Department of Veterans Affairs
Health Services Research & Development Service | Evidence-based Synthesis Program

Comparison of Quality of Care in VA and Non-VA Settings: A Systematic Review

September 2010

Prepared for:
Department of Veterans Affairs
Veterans Health Administration
Health Services Research & Development Service
Washington, DC 20420

Prepared by:
Evidence-based Synthesis Program (ESP) Center
West Los Angeles VA Medical Center
Los Angeles, CA
Paul G. Shekelle, MD, PhD, Director

Investigators:
Principal Investigators:
  Paul G. Shekelle, MD, PhD
  Steven Asch, MD, MPH

Co-Investigators:
  Peter Glassman, MBBS, MSc
  Sierra Matula, MD
  Amal Trivedi, MD, MPH

Research Associate:
  Isomi Miake-Lye, BA

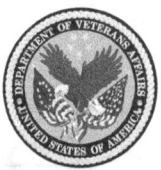

PREFACE

HSR&D's Evidence-based Synthesis Program (ESP) was established to provide timely and accurate syntheses of targeted healthcare topics of particular importance to VA managers and policymakers, as they work to improve the health and healthcare of Veterans. The ESP disseminates these reports throughout VA.

HSR&D provides funding for four ESP Centers and each Center has an active VA affiliation. The ESP Centers generate evidence syntheses on important clinical practice topics, and these reports help:

- develop clinical policies informed by evidence,
- the implementation of effective services to improve patient outcomes and to support VA clinical practice guidelines and performance measures, and
- set the direction for future research to address gaps in clinical knowledge.

In 2009, an ESP Coordinating Center was created to expand the capacity of HSR&D Central Office and the four ESP sites by developing and maintaining program processes. In addition, the Center established a Steering Committee comprised of HSR&D field-based investigators, VA Patient Care Services, Office of Quality and Performance, and VISN Clinical Management Officers. The Steering Committee provides program oversight and guides strategic planning, coordinates dissemination activities, and develops collaborations with VA leadership to identify new ESP topics of importance to Veterans and the VA healthcare system.

Comments on this evidence report are welcome and can be sent to Nicole Floyd, ESP Coordinating Center Program Manager, at nicole.floyd@va.gov.

Recommended citation:
Asch, S, Glassman P, Matula S, Trivedi A, Miake-Lye I and Shekelle P. Comparison of Quality of Care in VA and Non-VA Settings: A Systematic Review. VA-ESP Project # 05-226; 2010.

This report is based on research conducted by the Evidence-based Synthesis Program (ESP) Center located at the West Los Angeles VA Medical Center, Los Angeles, CA funded by the Department of Veterans Affairs, Veterans Health Administration, Office of Research and Development, Health Services Research and Development. The findings and conclusions in this document are those of the author(s) who are responsible for its contents; the findings and conclusions do not necessarily represent the views of the Department of Veterans Affairs or the United States government. Therefore, no statement in this article should be construed as an official position of the Department of Veterans Affairs. No investigators have any affiliations or financial involvement (e.g., employment, consultancies, honoraria, stock ownership or options, expert testimony, grants or patents received or pending, or royalties) that conflict with material presented in the report.

TABLE OF CONTENTS

EXECUTIVE SUMMARY iv
    Background iv
    Methods iv
    Results iv
    Conclusions vi

INTRODUCTION 1
    Background 1

METHODS 1
    Topic Development 1
    Search Strategy 1
    Study Selection 1
    Data Abstraction 2
    Quality Assessment 2
    Data Synthesis 2
    Peer Review 2

RESULTS 3
    Literature Flow 3
    Description of Evidence 4
    Surgical Conditions 4
        General Surgery 5
        Solid Organ Transplantation 6
        Vascular Surgery 8
        Surgical Oncology 9
        Cardiac Surgery 11
        Endocrine Surgery 12
    Medical and Other Non-Surgical Conditions 13
        General 13
        Cardiovascular 15
        Diabetes 17
        Hospital and Nursing Home Care 18
        Mental Health 19
        Other Studies 20

SUMMARY AND DISCUSSION 22
    Limitations 22
        Publication Bias 22
        Study Quality 22
    Conclusions 23
    Future Research 25

REFERENCES 27

FIGURES
    Figure 1 Literature Flow 4

APPENDICES
    Appendix 1. Evidence Table of Surgical Studies 32
    Appendix 2. Evidence Table of Medical and Non-surgical Studies 38
    Appendix 3. Screener Form 51
    Appendix 4. Data Abstraction Form 53
    Appendix 5. Data Abstraction Grading Guidelines 54
    Appendix 6. Search Strategy 55
    Appendix 7. Peer Review Comments Table 55

EXECUTIVE SUMMARY

BACKGROUND

It remains unclear where the Veterans Health Administration (VA) finds itself in the spectrum of care currently available in the United States. The quality of care provided by the VA has been subject to debate since, and well before, the VA's system transformation starting in the mid-90s. Media and entertainment vehicles have, rightly or wrongly, not infrequently portrayed VA care in less than optimal light, although there have been notable exceptions[1]. Regardless of media views, the VA has established itself as an innovative healthcare system, including implementation of its advanced electronic medical record, with broad clinical and educational missions.

The immediate objective of this project is to conduct a systematic literature review of the published literature comparing the quality of medical and surgical care provided by the VA to relevant non-VA healthcare facilities and systems.

The Key Question was:
Compare and contrast studies that assess VA and non-VA quality of care for surgical, non-surgical and other medical conditions.

METHODS

We were first given a list of articles by VA Central Office that represented examples of articles addressing possible VA and non-VA comparisons. Once these were reviewed, we then completed a Medline search for similar types of articles. Between the initial list and the subsequent search, we retrieved 222 articles. These were then screened by two physicians trained in the critical analysis of literature. Articles that both agreed were to be included were then reviewed, and all data were narratively summarized. When differences in the initial assessment (inclusion vs not) occurred, the specific articles were then discussed with at least one other senior member of the review team.

RESULTS

Of the 222 articles, mentioned above, 175 unique articles were identified and screened. Of these, 98 articles were initially rejected because there was no comparison of quality in VA and non-VA settings in the United States. After 22 articles were excluded because the comparisons were found to be non-contemporaneous, or had unequal or unrepresentative samples, used dissimilar or indirect measures of quality, had methodological problems, or were published before 1990 (which was used as an a priori cut off point), our first data abstraction included 55 articles. The 55 articles were categorized as either addressing surgical conditions (n=17) or medical and other non-surgical conditions (n=38).

Surgical Conditions

Ten of the seventeen articles, or more than half the available studies, came from the Patient Safety and Surgery Study, which was performed between 2001 and 2004, and grew out of collaboration between the American College of Sugeons and VA's National Surgical Quality Improvement Program.

Of four general surgery studies, three revealed no significant differences in adjusted postoperative morbidity rates while one found significantly lower rates of postoperative morbidity in the VA setting compared with the private sector. Three of the four studies assessed risk adjusted mortality rates and of these, two found no significant difference across settings. One study found significantly higher risk adjusted rates of postoperative mortality among male patients at the VA compared with the private sector. All four of these studies were part of the Patient Safety in Surgery Study.

Of three solid organ transplant articles, two found no significant differences in patient survival when comparing VA patients with non-VA patients. Additionally, one of these found no significant difference in graft survival between these two groups. This study also included a sub-analysis of health related quality of life (HRQOL) among heart and liver transplant recipients and found no significant difference in functional status or mental component scoring, but noted a trend toward lower physical component scores among VA patients by 7 years post-transplant. One study found that compared with privately insured patients, VA patients with end-stage renal disease were both less likely to be listed for a kidney transplant and less likely to receive a transplant when listed.

Of the three vascular surgery studies, two found significantly lower risk adjusted rates of postoperative morbidity in the VA and one found no significant difference in morbidity rates. There were no significant differences in risk adjusted mortality rates throughout these three studies. Two of the three vascular surgery studies were part of the Patient Safety in Surgery Study.

Of the three studies pertaining to surgical oncology, two focused on pancreatic cancer and one focused on breast cancer. One of the pancreatic cancer studies based on the National Cancer Data Base (NCDB) found no significant difference in postoperative mortality. The other study on pancreatic cancer based on the Patient Safety in Surgery Study found increased risk adjusted postoperative rates of morbidity and mortality in VA. The breast cancer study found no significant difference in risk adjusted postoperative morbidity among female patients. Two of the three surgical oncology studies came from the Patient Safety in Surgery Study (one pancreatic cancer study, one breast cancer study).

Two articles pertained to cardiac surgery. Of these, one focused on patient perceptions of numerous aspects of patient care after coronary artery bypass grafting in VA and non-VA hospitals. This study found that, after risk adjustment, VA patients were more likely than non-VA patients to report a problem with patient care. The second article compared severity adjusted mortality rates after CABG among VA and non-VA hospitals. After adjusting for patient-level predictors and hospital volume, the study found that the odds of death were higher in VA patients than in private sector patients.

In both of the endocrine surgery studies, there were no significant differences in postoperative morbidity or adverse event rates. Both endocrine surgery studies came out of the Patient Safety in Surgery Study.

Medical and Other Non-surgical Conditions

Of 10 general comparative studies assessing use of preventive services, acute and chronic care for multiple medical acute and chronic medical conditions, changes in broad health status including risk-adjusted morality, and patient satisfaction, each showed superior performance, as measured by greater adherence to accepted processes of care, better health outcomes or improved patient ratings of care, for care delivered in the VA compared with care delivered outside the VA. The studies used data from 1995 to 2004.

Of the 6 studies that assessed cardiovascular outcomes, 5 studies of mortality following an acute myocardial infarction or percutaneous coronary transluminal angioplasty found no clear survival differences between VA and non-VA settings and one study found greater control of blood pressure in the VA. Of the 3 studies that assessed use of processes of care following an acute myocardial infarction, all three found greater rates of evidence-based drug therapy in VA, and one study found lower use of clinically-appropriate angiography in the VA. Of note, all of these cardiovascular studies use data that are between 7 to 18 years old.

Four studies of the quality of diabetes care demonstrate a performance advantage on some measures for the VA compared with commercial managed care and other non-VA populations.

Studies of the quality of hospital and nursing home care demonstrate similar risk-adjusted mortality rates in VA facilities compared with non-VA facilities. VA hospitals had somewhat better patient safety outcomes compared with non-VA hospitals. Veterans in VA nursing homes were less likely to develop a pressure ulcer but more likely to experience functional decline compared to veterans in community nursing homes. In addition, the VA had higher use of infection control practices, but greater readmission rates and equivalent racial mortality differences.

Studies of the quality of mental health care demonstrate that the quality of antidepressant prescribing is slightly better in VA compared to private sector settings. One study of national data found VA patients with schizophrenia were more likely to receive an antipsychotic medication in the outpatient setting, but a study of data from two states found VA outpatients were less likely to receive an antipsychotic medication and psychosocial services. Among patients discharged after a hospitalization for schizophrenia, readmission and outpatient visit follow-up rates were worse in the VA, but continuity of care was better compared to the private sector.

Elderly VA patients were less likely to be prescribed potentially inappropriate medications than elderly patients in Medicare managed care plans. A study of survival following a diagnosis of lung carcinoma in Pennsylvania found worse survival for VA patients in that state. Stroke patients receiving rehabilitation in VA settings were discharged with better functional outcomes. VA patients had greater satisfaction with hearing aid fittings and somewhat greater self-reported benefit from hearing aid placement.

CONCLUSIONS

Overall, the available literature suggests that the care provided in the VA compares favorably to non-VA care systems, albeit with some caveats. Studies that used accepted process of care measures and intermediate outcomes measures, such as control of blood pressure or hemoglobin A1c, for quality measurements almost always found VA performed better than non-VA comparison groups. Studies looking at risk-adjusted outcomes generally have found no differences between VA and non-VA care, with some reports of better outcomes in VA and a few reports of worse outcomes in VA, compared to non-VA care. The studies of processes of care are mostly those about medical conditions, while the studies of outcomes are mostly about surgical conditions and interventional procedures.

INTRODUCTION

BACKGROUND

As noted by Ashton et al, VA healthcare system transformation began in 1995, moving from a hospital-based system to a more comprehensive healthcare model with the goal of providing the best health care in America[2]. There have been numerous reports comparing VA health care quality with non-VA care, both scholarly and in the lay media[1, 3-5]. However, there has not been a systematic evaluation of the published evidence comparing care across systems. Therefore, VA Central Office asked the Evidence Synthesis Program located at the VA Greater Los Angeles Healthcare System, West Los Angeles campus to perform such a review.

METHODS

TOPIC DEVELOPMENT

This project was nominated by William Duncan, Associate Deputy Undersecretary of Health for Quality and Safety.

The final key question was:

Compare and contrast studies that assess VA and non-VA quality of care for surgical, non-surgical and other medical conditions.

SEARCH STRATEGY

We were first given a list of articles by VA Central Office that represented examples of articles addressing possible VA and non-VA comparisons. Once these were reviewed, we then completed a Medline search for similar types of articles. Between the initial list and the subsequent search, we retrieved 222 articles. These were then screened by two physicians trained in the critical analysis of literature. Articles that both agreed were to be included were then reviewed, and all data were narratively summarized. When differences in the initial assessment (inclusion vs not) occurred, the specific articles were then discussed with at least one other senior member of the review team. Because of the focus on US health care, we searched Medline only. The search strategy is listed in Appendix 6.

STUDY SELECTION

Articles were reviewed utilizing a two page screening form (see Appendix 3). Each article was reviewed by two physicians, one with a surgical background and the other specializing in internal medicine. To be included in our report, the article had to present a comparison of quality of clinical data in VA and United States (US) non-VA settings, and had to have been published no earlier than 1990. The screening form also collected basic information about the articles: whether or not the data for the comparison was sufficiently contemporaneous (within 1 to 2 years of each other); how VA and non-VA data were assembled; from what geographical area(s) VA and non-VA data were collected and analyzed; what conditions were covered in the quality assessment;

what features of quality were measured (structure, process, and/or outcomes); and how similar were the specifications for the quality assessments comparing VA and non-VA samples.

DATA ABSTRACTION

Data were independently abstracted using a one-page abstraction form (see Appendix 4). Data for surgically related articles were abstracted by our surgical reviewer, and for non-surgical articles the internal medicine reviewer completed the abstraction process. Once the forms were completed, all data were reviewed by the review team. The following data were abstracted from included trials: sample size for both VA and non-VA sources, years of data collection covered for both VA and non-VA sources; control variables; primary outcomes; and secondary or associated findings.

QUALITY ASSESSMENT

Each article was given an overall assessment, which was based on the following criteria: time frames; samples (both VA and non-VA); quality measurements; outcomes; importance of measures; and statistical methods. Each of these factors was assigned a grade (A, B, or C) based on the data abstraction grading guidelines developed (see Appendix 5). The overall assessment was predicated on the global assessment of the article, considering the individual components, but was not an average. Thus an article that had, for example, a critical flaw in methodology would be a "C," even if other issues were satisfactory. During this phase, or during the initial assessment or data abstraction phases, disagreements or questions about the articles or information were discussed with at least one senior member of the team in order to reach concurrence.

DATA SYNTHESIS

We first classified articles as dealing with surgical or medical therapy. Within these categories, we further grouped articles according to their clinical content area, for example, one group contained medical studies about the quality of cardiovascular disease care. Within these categories, studies were still sufficiently heterogenous to preclude meta-analysis. Consequently, our synthesis is narrative.

PEER REVIEW

A draft version of this report was sent to six peer reviewers, of which one responded. Her comments and our responses are presented in Appendix 7. Peer Review Comments Table.

RESULTS

LITERATURE FLOW

In total, we examined 222 articles, from the "VHA Clinical Quality and Patient Safety: A review of the medical literature" and our second systematic literature search.

Of the titles identified in the review, 47 articles were rejected as duplicates. This left 175 articles to be screened.

From this initial screening, 98 articles were rejected because there was no comparison of quality in VA and US non-VA settings. Four more articles were rejected for falling before the cutoff date of 1990. Our data abstraction thus included 73 articles, 18 of which were rejected, having received a grade of C or having failed to meet the initial inclusion criteria upon further inspection.

Upon categorization, these final 55 articles were divided between surgical articles (n=17) and non-surgical/medical articles (n=38). Within the surgical category, there were 4 general surgury, 3 vascular surgery, 3 oncologic surgery, 3 solid organ transplantation, 2 cardiac surgery, and 2 endocrine articles. Within the medical category there were 10 general, 8 cardiovascular, 8 hospital care, 4 diabetes, 4 mental health care, and 4 other articles (See Figure 1).

Figure 1 Literature Flow

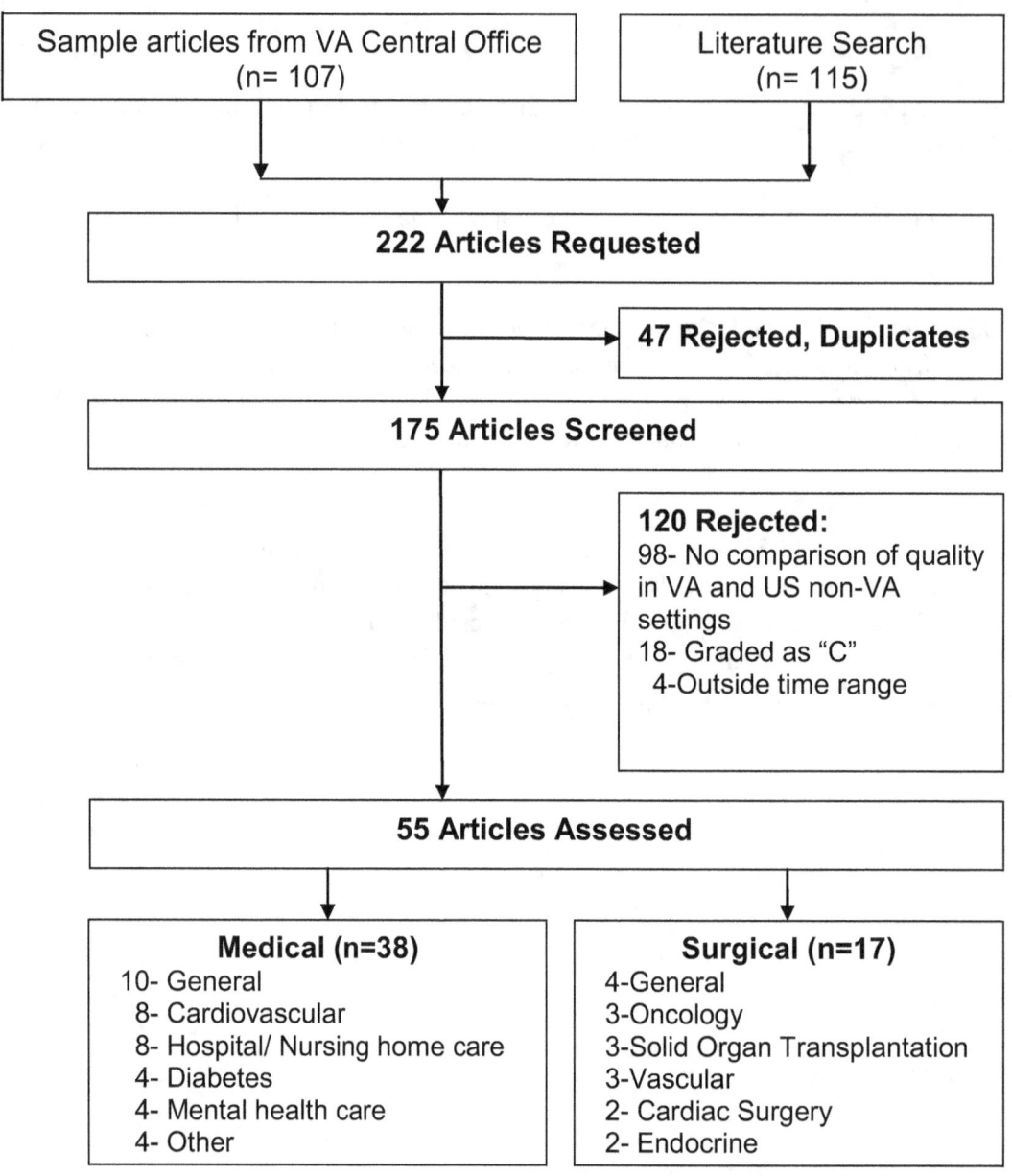

DESCRIPTION OF EVIDENCE

We evaluated studies that compared quality of care for medical and surgical conditions in the Veterans Health Administration (VA) with clinical care in settings outside the VA. We summarize these data in the next two sections.

SURGICAL CONDITIONS

We found 17 comparisons that met the inclusion criteria and pertained to the field of surgery[6-22]. Four of these addressed general surgery conditions[9, 13, 16, 17], three addressed solid organ transplantation[6, 10, 18], three addressed vascular surgery[14, 15, 22], three addressed surgical oncology[7, 11, 19], two addressed cardiac surgery[8, 20], and two addressed endocrine surgery[12, 21]. Ten of the seventeen articles came out of the Patient Safety in Surgery Study which was performed from October 1, 2001 through September 30, 2004[9, 11-17, 19, 21]. The Patient Safety in Surgery Study grew out of collaboration between the American College of Surgeons and the VA, and aimed to determine if implementation of the National Surgical Quality Improvement Program (NSQIP) in the private sector could reduce postoperative mortality and morbidity in non-VA settings. This study compared risk adjusted postoperative morbidity and mortality for a number of general and vascular surgical conditions between the VA system and 14 university medical centers that had volunteered to be early adopters of NSQIP.

GENERAL SURGERY

Four articles fell into the general surgery category[9, 13, 16, 17]; of these, two addressed general surgery broadly[9, 13], one addressed liver resections[16] and one addressed bariatric surgery[17]. All four of these articles were based on data from the Patient Safety in Surgery Study described above. The primary outcomes across studies were postoperative morbidity and mortality. Findings across these studies were heterogeneous.

Of the two broad general surgery papers, one focused on men and the other focused on women undergoing general surgery operations. Henderson and colleagues evaluated 94,098 general surgery operations in men at 128 VA medical centers and compared this with 18,399 general surgery operations in men in 14 university hospitals[13]. The main types of surgery performed were different in each population. Unadjusted postoperative morbidity and mortality rates were higher in the private sector compared with the VA. Stepwise logistic regression, adjusting for patient and disease characteristics, revealed no significant difference in postoperative morbidity across sites. However there were significantly greater odds of postoperative mortality in the VA (OR 1.23, 95% CI (1.08-1.41). Additional analysis revealed differences in unadjusted mortality rate by procedure type. Unadjusted mortality rates were comparable among the five most common general surgical operations performed in the VA and the private sector (open inguinal hernia, partial colectomy, laparoscopic cholecystectomy, umbilical hernia, ventral hernia), however unadjusted mortality rates were higher in the VA for less common, more complex operations (pancreatectomy, adrenalectomy, bariatric operation, thyroidectomy/parathyroidectomy and hepatectomy). Risk adjustments evaluated general surgery broadly and did not account for specific type of surgery.

Fink and colleagues reviewed 5,157 female patients in the VA and 27,367 female patients in the private sector who underwent general surgery operations during the Patient Safety in Surgery[9]. As in the study of male patients, certain procedures were performed more frequently in each of the two settings: more endocrine and laparoscopic procedures in the private sector and more lumpectomies and radical mastectomies in the VA. Unadjusted morbidity rates were higher in the private sector, likely attributable to the significantly higher incidence of urinary tract infections in this population. Unadjusted mortality rates were comparable across systems of care. After stepwise logistic regression to adjust for patient and disease characteristics there were significantly lower risk adjusted odds of developing a postoperative complication among the VA cohort compared with the private sector (OR 0.80, 95% CI 0.71-0.90); there was no significant difference in risk adjusted postoperative mortality among women undergoing general surgery operations. Risk adjustments evaluated general surgery broadly and did not account for specific type of surgery.

Lancaster and colleagues reviewed 237 VA and 783 private sector hepatectomies as part of the Patient Safety in Surgery Study[16]. Unadjusted morbidity and mortality rates were higher in the VA. After adjusting for pre-operative patient characteristics, lifestyle factors and intra-operative characteristics, morbidity and mortality rates were not significantly different between the VA and private sector university hospitals studied (morbidity 0.940, 95% CI 0.623-1.421and mortality OR 1.623, 95% CI 0.609-4.324).

Lautz and colleagues evaluated 374 patients who underwent bariatric surgery in 12 VA hospitals and 2,064 patients who underwent bariatric surgery in the 12 private sector hospitals as part of the Patient Safety in Surgery Study[17]. Male and female VA patients were significantly more likely to undergo an open operation, had surgeries with higher mean relative value units and were hospitalized longer than private sector patients. Unadjusted morbidity and mortality rates were comparable in women across cohorts. After risk adjustment, there were still no significant differences in postoperative morbidity among women in the VA versus private sector. Unadjusted and adjusted morbidity rates were higher among men treated at the VA compared with the private sector (adjusted OR 2.99, 95% CI 1.28-4.10). Unadjusted mortality rates were significantly higher among men treated at the VA compared with the private sector. There were too few deaths to allow for determination of risk adjusted rates.

Summary: Of four general surgery studies, three revealed no significant differences in adjusted postoperative morbidity rates while one found significantly lower rates of postoperative morbidity in the VA setting compared with the private sector. Three of the 4 studies assessed risk adjusted mortality rates and of these, two found no significant difference across settings. One study found significantly higher risk adjusted rates of postoperative mortality among male patients at the VA compared with the private sector.

SOLID ORGAN TRANSPLANTATION

Three articles addressed solid organ transplantation in VA and non-VA patients. Of these, one addressed orthotopic liver transplant only[6], one addressed renal transplantation[10], and one evaluated outcomes after liver, heart, renal and lung transplant[18]. Two studies compared survival. Of these, one evaluated mortality at one, three and five years post-OLT[6], and one evaluated graft survival and patient survival after heart, lung, kidney and liver transplant[18]. The latter study also evaluated health related quality of life as a secondary outcome. The final study assessed differences in time to renal transplantation[10].

Austin and colleagues studied 149 VA patients and 285 private sector patients who underwent orthotopic liver transplantation (OLT) at a single medical center between September 1991 and December 2000[6]. They aimed to determine whether there was a difference in mortality after OLT in US veterans compared with non-veterans and to evaluate what, if any, factors made a difference. Veterans received their pre and post transplant care at the Portland Veterans Affairs Medical Center (PVAMC) and non-Veterans received pre and post transplant care at the Oregon

Health and Science University hospital; however, all patients were transplanted in the operating rooms of the VA and received initial postoperative intensive care at the VA. The outcome of interest was mortality at one, three and five years post transplant. Veterans had increased mortality rates as assessed by Kaplan-Meier curves. After adjusting for gender, donor age, recipient age, etiology of liver disease and MELD score, hospital status was not a significant predictor of mortality RR 1.15 (95% CI 0.94-1.43). In multivariate analysis, donor age was most predictive of survival. Austin et al found no significant difference between patient groups when evaluating time spent on the waiting list between evaluation and treatment. At the time of initial evaluation, patients who were veterans had lower average serum albumin levels and a higher percentage of patients with Child's class C liver disease suggesting that perhaps veterans were referred later in the disease course. This study was limited in its retrospective nature, and in its inability to account for cause of death or account for pre transplant comorbidities. Additionally, use of the MELD score became standard during the course of the study, and thus the patient population included across this ten year time period may not be representative of patients who are eligible for or undergo transplant today. Due to missing data, 60 patients (43 university patients and 17 veterans) were excluded from the analyses. Five year survival was significantly different between the included and excluded patients overall (50% versus 73% respectively) potentially causing a bias in the results. Finally, this study was unable to account for post transplant substance abuse.

Moore et al were interested in comparing comprehensive outcomes in VA transplant patients compared with non-VA transplant patients[18]. They studied all adult patients from Vanderbilt University Medical Center and the VA Tennessee Valley Healthcare System who underwent a primary liver, kidney, heart or lung transplant between 1990 and 2002. All patients received heart, liver and lung transplants at VUMC; renal transplants were performed at both centers. VA patients received up to 3 months of postoperative care at VUMC prior to transfer back to the VA setting. Groups were distinguished primarily by payer status. Primary outcomes were graft survival and patient survival. Additionally, health related quality of life (HRQOL) was assessed in a subset of patients using Karnofsky functional performance and the SF-36. A total of 380 VA patients (141 liver, 54 heart, 183 kidney, 2 lung) were compared with 1,429 non-VA patients (280 liver, 246 heart, 749 kidney, 154 lung). Due to the limited number of lung transplant recipients, comparisons of outcomes were not performed in this subgroup. Cumulative graft survival was not significantly different between the two patient populations for liver transplant (p=0.97), heart transplant (p=0.67) or renal transplant (p=0.84). Similarly, cumulative patient survival was not significantly different between the two populations for liver (p=0.94, heart (p=0.75) or renal (p=0.12) transplant patients. HRQOL was assessed in a subset of 77 liver and 70 heart transplant recipients. Overall, there were significant improvements in functional performance from pre-transplant to 2 years post-transplant ((49+2 versus 90+2; (p<0.001. However, there was no significant difference in functional performance between VA and non-VA patients from the pre to post-transplant state (p=0.065). Additionally, there was no significant difference in functional performance between VA and non-VA patients at three (p=0.50) or seven years (p=0.17) post-transplant. SF-36 mental component scores measured post-transplant were not significantly different between the two patient populations. However, physical component scales diverged after 7 years post-transplant, with VA patients reporting slightly worse physical component scale (PCS) scores compared with non-VA patients (35+2 versus 39+1, p=0.05); mental component scale scores remained similar over time (47+2 versus 49+1, p=0.29 at 7 years post transplant). This study was limited in its cross sectional nature regarding HRQOL data; in addition, the patient populations were restricted to a single transplant program, potentially limiting the generalizability of the findings. Recurrence of hepatitis C and other patient level characteristics over time could not be taken into account, thus limiting ability to interpret the meaning behind the PCS scores long term. Additionally, the article does not make clear how the subset of heart and liver transplants was selected in order to evaluate HRQOL nor is the breakdown specified of VA and non-VA patients in this subset.

Gill et al used national data from the US Renal Data System from April 1, 1995 through December 31, 2004 to compare the time to transplantation among ESRD patients either covered by VA or insured by private insurance or Medicare/Medicaid[10]. A total of 7,395 VA patients were compared with 144,651 privately insured patients and an additional 357,345 insured by Medicare or Medicaid. After adjusting for patient demographics, clinical characteristics and state rates of transplantation, they found that VA-covered and Medicare/Medicaid-insured patients were approximately 35% less likely to receive transplants than patients with private insurance (hazard ratio [HR] 0.65; 95% CI 0.60 to 0.70; P < 0.0001). VA patients were less likely to be placed on the wait-list (HR 0.71; 95% CI 0.67 to 0.76). VA patients who were on the wait list also received transplants less frequently than privately insured patients (HR 0.89; 95% CI 0.82 to 0.96). VA patients with supplemental private insurance had the same likelihood of transplantation as non-VA patients with private insurance. Study limitations included unmeasured variables and inability to account for VA covered patients who had access to transplantation outside of the VA.

Summary: Of three solid organ transplant articles, two found no significant differences in patient survival when comparing VA patients with non-VA patients. Additionally, one of these found no significant difference in graft survival between these two groups. This study also included a sub-analysis of health related quality of life (HRQOL) among heart and liver transplant recipients and found no significant difference in functional status or mental component scoring, but noted a trend toward lower physical component scores among VA patients by 7 years post-transplant. One study found that compared with privately insured patients, VA patients with end-stage renal disease were both less likely to be listed for a kidney transplant and less likely to receive a transplant when listed.

VASCULAR SURGERY

Three studies compared quality of care in the VA and the private sector in vascular surgery[14, 15, 22]. Two were from the Patient Safety in Surgery Study looking at male and female patients respectively[14, 15]. Hutter and colleagues evaluated 30,058 operations in men in the VA and 5174 in the private sector as part of the Patient Safety in Surgery Study[14]. The two populations had significantly different preoperative risk profiles. There were significantly different types and frequencies of vascular surgeries in the groups; for example, there were more carotid endarterectomies in the VA and more open abdominal aortic aneurysm repairs in the private sector. Unadjusted postoperative morbidity and mortality rates were higher in the private sector. After stepwise logistic regression adjusting for preoperative and intraoperative variables there was a significantly lower odds of perioperative complications in the VA (OR 0.84, 95% CI 0.78-0.92). There was no significant difference in risk adjusted mortality between the VA and private sector (p=0.195), although it was not clear how the relevant indicator variable for system of care was used in the model.

Johnson and colleagues used data from the Patient Safety in Surgery Study to compare 458 female VA patients and 3,535 non-VA female patients who underwent vascular surgery[15]. The two populations differed across many categories in assessing preoperative risk profile with private sector patients having a greater incidence of various preoperative morbidities. Private sector vascular operations were more likely to be emergencies. Types and frequencies of vascular surgery operations differed considerably across hospital type. For example VA patients had carotid endarterectomies, saphenous vein ligation and arteriovenous fistulas more commonly than private sector patients; private sector patients underwent above the knee amputations, femoral popliteal bypass with artificial graft material, femorotibial bypass and open abdominal aortic aneurysm more frequently than VA patients. Unadjusted postoperative morbidity and mortality were higher in the private sector. After stepwise logistic regression adjusting for patient and intra-operative characteristics, there was no significant difference in 30 day mortality rates among VA and PS female vascular patients; there was a significantly lower odds of experiencing a postoperative complication among VA patients compared with private sector patients (OR 0.60, 05%CI 0.44-0.81). Both the Hutter and Johnson studies were unable to account for endovascular procedures performed outside the operating room (such as in the radiology or cardiology suites).

Weiss and colleagues evaluated perioperative mortality, stroke and cardiac complications in patients undergoing carotid endarterectomy in Connecticut from October 1997-September [22]. VA data was derived from the Connecticut VA database that comprised data submitted to the VA-NSQIP. Private sector data was derived from the Connecticut Hospital Association database. They evaluated 140 carotid endarterectomies in the VA setting and 6,949 CEAs in the private sector. Based on a modified Charlson comorbidity score, patients in the VA had higher comorbidities than patients in the private sector. Unadjusted rates of mortality, stroke and cardiac complications were higher in the VA, though these differences were not significant. After adjusting for patient and disease characteristics, there were no significant differences in postoperative mortality, stroke or rate of cardiac complications. This study was limited by the small sample size and narrow geographic region and thus may not be generalizable to other VA or private sector settings. Additionally, the data sources were different for each cohort with VA data taken from NSQIP which includes chart abstraction while private sector data were derived from inpatient registries.

Summary: Of the three vascular surgery studies, two found significantly lower risk adjusted rates of postoperative morbidity in the VA and one found no significant difference in morbidity rates. There were no significant differences in risk adjusted mortality rates throughout these three studies.

SURGICAL ONCOLOGY

Of the three articles on surgical oncology[7, 11, 19], two focused on pancreatic cancer[7, 11] and one focused on breast cancer[19]. The pancreatic cancer papers were derived from two data sources. Bilimoria and colleagues used the National Cancer Data Base (NCDB) to evaluate 513 VA patients, 12,576 academic hospital patients and 18,299 community hospital patients who underwent treatment for stage I and II pancreatic cancer from 1985-2004[7]. The cohorts differed significantly in the distributions of age, gender, race, disease stage, income, insurance and

Charlson comorbidity score. The outcomes assessed included 60 day and 3 year mortality, as well as stage appropriate treatment including receipt of neoadjuvant therapy and resection. After adjusting for patient, surgical, disease and hospital characteristics, they found that mortality rates were comparable between the VA, academic and community hospital settings for resection of stage I and II pancreatic cancer. After risk adjustment, there was no difference in use of surgery or adjuvant chemotherapy between VA and academic hospitals (p=0.54), however VA hospitals were significantly more likely to use surgery and adjuvant chemotherapy than community hospitals (p<0.001). The use of NCDB only accounts for hospitals accredited by the American College of Surgeons Commission on Cancer thus there is a potential selection bias; additionally, this limits the generalizability of the findings to participating centers. Comorbidity data was only available through the NCDB starting in 2003, thus risk adjustment on patient characteristics was limited to the tail end of the study period. Finally, the reference group in the analyses was the VA which was also the smallest sample size.

The second article on pancreatic cancer was by Glasgow and colleagues; they used the Patient Safety in Surgery Study to compare postoperative morbidity and mortality after pancreatectomy for pancreatic cancer at 83 VA hospitals and 14 private sector hospitals[11]. Three hundred and seventy seven VA patients and 692 private sector patients were included. There were considerable differences in preoperative comorbidity profiles across cohorts. VA patients were less likely to be admitted from home and more likely to receive a blood transfusion intraoperatively. Using stepwise logistic regression to adjust for case mix differences, patient characteristics and intra-operative variables, they found higher rates of both 30 day postoperative morbidity (OR 1.58, 95% CI 1.08-2.31) and mortality (OR 2.53, 95% CI 1.02-2.38) in the VA compared with the private sector. These findings persisted after stratifying analyses by Whipple procedure or pancreaticoduodenectomy.

The final article pertaining to surgical oncology was done by Neumayer and colleagues as part of the Patient Safety in Surgery Study to compare postoperative morbidity from breast cancer surgery in the VA and private sector[19]. There were 644 VA patients and 3,179 private sector patients identified. The majority of the patients were female (n=3,634) and results were stratified by gender. Both male and female VA patients had more preoperative comorbidities, higher rates of mastectomy and higher unadjusted complication rates than their private sector counterparts. Stepwise logistic regression was done in the female cohort, adjusting for patient factors, disease characteristics, surgeon traits and type of surgery. There was no significant difference in risk adjusted 30 day morbidity between female patients in the VA and private sector (OR 1.40, 95% CI 0.89-2.20). Risk adjusted outcomes were not reported for the male cohort of breast cancer patients.

Summary: Of the three studies pertaining to surgical oncology, two focused on pancreatic cancer and one focused on breast cancer. One of the pancreatic cancer studies based on the National Cancer Data Base (NCDB) found no significant difference in postoperative mortality. The other study on pancreatic cancer based on the Patient Safety in Surgery Study found increased risk adjusted postoperative rates of morbidity and mortality in VA. The breast cancer study found no significant difference in risk adjusted postoperative morbidity among female patients. Two of the three surgical oncology studies came from the Patient Safety in Surgery Study (one pancreatic cancer study, one breast cancer study).

CARDIAC SURGERY

Two articles pertained to cardiac surgery[8, 20]. Of these, one focused on patient perceptions of numerous aspects of patient care after coronary artery bypass grafting in VA and non-VA hospitals[8]. The second article compared severity adjusted mortality rates after CABG among VA and non-VA hospitals[20].

Feria et al compared perceptions of aspects of patient care among male patients undergoing coronary artery bypass graft (CABG) in both VA and non-VA settings between 1995 and 1998[8]. The domains of patient care that were examined included respect for patient preferences, emotional support, patient education and communication, coordination of care, concern for physical comfort, family participation, transition to discharge, access, and courtesy. The VA sample consisted of 808 patients who underwent CABG at 43 VA hospitals. Perceptions were evaluated in postoperative surveys collected through the VA National Performance Feedback Center. The non-VA sample consisted of 2271 patients who underwent CABG at 102 non-VA hospitals. Data were extracted from routine postoperative surveys by the Picker Institute; hospitals were included only if they had contracted with the Picker Institute. After controlling for age, race, self-reported health status, and diagnosis related group, VA patients were more likely than non-VA patients to note a problem with patient care in 8 of the 9 dimensions with the exception of transition to discharge ($p<0.001$). Adjusted differences in the percentage of questions for which VA patients reported a problem relative to non-VA patients were significant in these 8 domains, including access (3.2, 95% CI 1.5-4.8), coordination of care (4.8, 95% CI 3.0-6.6), courtesy (2,9, 95% CI 1.4-4.5), patient education and information (7.1, 95% CI 4.4-9.8), emotional support (5.5, 95% CI 2.7-8.3), family participation (5.5, 95% CI 2.3-8.7), concern for physical comfort and(3.9, 95% CI 2.3-5.5) respect for patient preferences (6.2, 95% CI 3.6-8.7). A sub-analysis limited to teaching hospital settings found that VA patients remained more likely to note a problem with care in 5 dimensions including coordination of care, courtesy, patient education and information, emotional support and concern for physical comfort. Adjusted differences in percentage of questions for which VA patients reported a problem relative to non-VA patients were significant across 7 of the 9 dimensions of care including access (2.7, 95% CI 0.4-5.3), coordination of care (4.1, 95% CI 1.3-6.9), courtesy (2,3, 95% CI 0.5-4.2), patient education and information (6.0, 95% CI 2.9-9.1), emotional support (4.0 95% CI 0.9-7.1), concern for physical comfort and(3.0, 95% CI 1.2-4.8) respect for patient preferences (5.1, 95% CI 2.2-8.0). Limitations to this study included the many unmeasured variables, such as socioeconomic status, education level, literacy, patient autonomy in selecting providers, type and severity of comorbidities, emergency or elective surgery and hospital size and location. The non-VA sample was limited to hospitals contracting with the Picker Institute which accounted for only about 9% of US non-VA hospitals; the overall analysis was limited to a male population. Given these issues, the results may not be generalizable.

Rosenthal et al compared severity adjusted mortality after CABG among VA hospitals and private sector in two geographic regions between October 1993 and December 1996[20]. They studied 19,266 patients from 43 VA hospitals using data from the VA Continuous Improvement in Cardiac Surgery Program. An additional 44,247 patients from 32 New York state hospitals were studied using data from the New York State Cardiac Surgery Reporting System and 9,696 patients from 10 hospitals in the northeast Ohio were studied using data from the Cleveland

Health Quality Choice. Each of these well established data sources contains slightly different information pertaining to patient and disease related traits; the VA CICSP contains about 90 components; the Cleveland Health Quality Choice collects about 250 items and the NY State Cardiac Surgery Reporting System collects data on 100 elements. VA patients were more likely to have congestive heart failure, chronic obstructive pulmonary disease, cerebrovascular disease, peripheral vascular disease and diabetes requiring medication than private sector patients. After adjusting for patient-level predictors and hospital volume, the study found that the odds of death were higher in VA patients than in private sector patients (OR, 1.34; 95% CI, 1.11-1.63; P <0.001). When comparing VA patients with those from NY State hospitals, a similar difference was found. However the comparison between VA and Northeast Ohio hospitals did not find a statistically significant difference in mortality rates. After stratifying by hospital volume, the odds of death among hospitals that performed 500 to 1000 CABG procedures annually were higher in VA hospitals than in private hospitals (OR 1.50, 95% CI 1.16-1.92, p=0.002) though this was not noted for lower CABG volumes (i.e., < 500) Limitations of this study included dependence on administrative data, unmeasured variable bias, potential systematic differences in data collection by the three data repositories used and geographic limitations to comparison groups potentially limiting generalizability of the findings. Additionally, the study period of 1993 to1996 may not represent current outcomes or performance.

Summary: Two articles pertained to cardiac surgery. Of these, one focused on patient perceptions of numerous aspects of patient care after coronary artery bypass grafting in VA and non-VA hospitals. This study found that, after risk adjustment, VA patients were more likely than non-VA patients to report a problem with patient care. The second article compared severity adjusted mortality rates after CABG among VA and non-VA hospitals. After adjusting for patient-level predictors and hospital volume, the study found that the odds of death were higher in VA patients than in private sector patients.

ENDOCRINE SURGERY

Two articles addressed issues in endocrine surgery[12, 21]. Each of these was from the Patient Safety in Surgery Study. One looked at 30 day postoperative morbidity and mortality after adrenalectomy[21], the other looked at the same outcomes after thyroidectomy or parathyroidectomy[12]. Turrentine and colleagues evaluated 178 patients in 81 VA hospitals and 371 patients in 14 private sector hospitals who underwent adrenalectomy[21]. VA patients were more likely to be older, male and to have greater preoperative risk profiles. VA operations were less likely to be laparoscopic. Unadjusted morbidity and mortality rates were higher in the VA compared with the private sector, however after adjusting for patient characteristics (including demographics, comorbidities, lab values), provider characteristics and wound class, there was no significant difference in postoperative morbidity among VA patients compared with private sector patients (OR 1.55, 95% CI 0.49-1.36). The mortality rate was too low for adjustment.

Hall and colleagues used the Patient Safety in Surgery Study to evaluate 2,814 VA patients and 4,268 patients in the private sector who underwent thyroidectomy or parathyroidectomy[12]. There were significantly different distributions of types of surgery at different sites with proportionally more parathyroid operations done at the VA. Unadjusted morbidity and mortality rates were significantly higher in the VA. Because the event rates for morbidity and mortality were very low, a combined variable was built for an outcome of 'any adverse event'. Stepwise logistic regression evaluated adverse event rates, accounting for disease type, surgical specialty and patient characteristics. Risk adjusted adverse event rates did not differ significantly across sites (OR 1.25, 95% CI 0.87-1.78).

Summary: In both of the endocrine studies, there were no significant differences in postoperative morbidity or adverse event rates.

MEDICAL AND OTHER NON-SURGICAL CONDITIONS

We identified 38 studies that compared quality of care for medical or other non-surgical conditions in the VA with clinical care in settings outside the VA[23-54 26, 55-57 25, 27, 58-61]. Of these, 10 studies (classified into a "general" category) assessed primary preventive services, multiple medical conditions, health status (including risk-adjusted mortality), or patient satisfaction [23, 28-30, 32, 40-42, 45, 46]; 8 studies assessed cardiovascular conditions[24, 34-36, 38, 47-49]; 4 studies assessed diabetes[31, 39, 50, 51]; 8 studies assessed hospital and nursing home care[33, 37, 43, 44, 53, 54, 60, 61]; 4 studies assessed mental health care[26, 55-57]; and 4 studies assessed other conditions[25, 27, 58, 59].

GENERAL

We identified 3 studies of preventive services and all found substantially higher rates of influenza and pneumococcal vaccination for the elderly in the VA compared to samples drawn from outside the VA[28, 30, 32]. These studies rely on self-reported survey data from the Medicare Current Beneficiary Survey (MCBS) and the Behavioral Risk Factor Surveillance System (BRFSS). The MCBS, sponsored by the Centers for Medicare and Medicaid Services, is a survey of the health status, health care utilization, and demographic characteristics of a nationally-representative sample of aged, disabled, or institutionalized Medicare beneficiaries. The BRFSS, sponsored by the Centers for Disease Control and Prevention, is an annual state-based system of health surveys that collects information on the health risk behaviors, preventive health practices, and health care access of a nationally representative sample of nearly 350,000 adults.

Keyhani et al. used data from the 2000 to 2003 MCBS to examine use of pneumococcal and influenza vaccination and serum cholesterol screening among veterans age 65 and older using the VA exclusively compared to veterans age 65 and older using the Medicare fee-for-service and the Medicare managed care programs[32]. In this study, veterans using the VA reported 10% greater use of influenza vaccination (P< 0.05), 14% greater use of pneumococcal vaccination (P< 0.01), and a non-significant 6% greater use of serum cholesterol screening (P= 0.1), than did veterans receiving care through Medicare HMOs. Veterans receiving care through the Medicare fee-for-service program reported lower use of all three of these preventive services compared to veterans using the VA.

Jha et al. also assessed rates of vaccination using quality of care data abstracted from VA medical records among persons 65 and older in the VA compared to a similar age group of community-dwelling persons responding to the BRFSS[30]. Influenza and pneumonia vaccination rates were significantly greater in the VA compared to those reported in the BRFSS. In 2003, the absolute differences between the VA and the community based sample were approximately 10 percentage points for influenza vaccination and 30 percentage points for pneumococcal vaccination. The study was limited by non-equivalent methods of assessment of vaccination; chart review was used in the VA sample and self-report was used in the non-VA sample.

Finally, Chi et al used data from the 2003 BRFSS to assess influenza and pneumonia vaccination rates for veterans using the VA, veterans not using the VA, and non-veterans[28]. They found that for both influenza and pneumococcal vaccination, veterans using the VA had higher vaccination rates than both veterans not using the VA and non-veterans. Compared to veterans not using the VA, veterans using the VA had an 8 percentage point greater adjusted rate of receiving an influenza vaccination (72% vs. 80%, P < 0.001)) and a 17 percentage point greater rate of receiving pneumococcal vaccination (64% vs. 81%, P < 0.001)

We identified 3 studies that compared quality of care for multiple acute and chronic medical conditions[23, 29, 40]. Jha et al. compared quality of care in the VA and Medicare fee-for-service using 13 equivalent process of care measures[29]. The study assessed care for patients with diabetes, acute myocardial infarction, and congestive heart failure using data from the VA's External Peer Review Program (EPRP), a previously published study of Medicare quality, and the Behavioral Risk Factor Surveillance System. The VA had statistically significant greater performance rates than the Medicare fee-for-service program on all 11 similar indicators from 1997 to 1999 and of 12 of 13 indicators in 2000. The exception was eye exams for patients with diabetes. In 2000, the VA equaled or exceeded 90% on 8 of 13 indicators while Medicare's highest performance on any indicator was 84%.

Asch et al. assessed clinical performance on over 300 process of care indicators in a sample of 596 VA patients in 2 VISNs and a random sample of 992 adults from 12 communities that were selected to be representative of non-rural communities in the United States[23]. The authors found that, overall, VA patients were more likely than patients in the national sample to receive the care specified by the indicators (67% vs. 51%; difference, 16 percentage points [CI, 14 to 18 percentage points]). The VA outperformed the non-VA sample for both chronic care (72% vs. 59%; difference, 13 percentage points [CI, 10 to 17 percentage points]) and preventive care (64% vs. 44%; difference, 20 percentage points [CI, 12 to 28 percentage points]), but not for acute care. The biggest difference was in performance measures targeted by the VA (adjusted scores, 67% vs. 43%; difference, 24 percentage points [CI, 21 to 26 percentage points]).

Finally, Ross et al. compared self-reported use of 17 preventive services for cancer prevention, cardiovascular risk reduction, diabetes mellitus management, and infectious disease prevention among insured adults receiving and not receiving care in the VA[40]. The data were derived from the 2000 and 2004 BRFSS. The study found that in 2000, persons receiving VAMC care were more likely to receive 6 of the 17 services; in 2004, persons receiving VAMC care reported greater use of 12 of the 17 services. In 2004, the performance advantage for the VA among these 12 services ranged from 10% greater use of cholesterol screening to 40% greater use of colorectal cancer screening. In 2004, there were no services for which rates of use were significantly greater for insured populations outside the VA than for patients using the VA.

We identified 3 studies that assessed changes in risk adjusted mortality and health status for elderly VA patients compared to elderly patients enrolled in Medicare Advantage (MA) plans[41, 42, 46]. Selim et al. surveyed a cohort of VA and MA enrollees at baseline and then 2 years later using the Short Form 36, a validated measure of health status[42]. They also linked these surveys to the death master file to assess status. In analyses adjusting for demographic characteristics, clinical conditions, and baseline health status, MA enrollees had a greater risk of 2 year mortality compared to VA patients (9.2% vs. 7.5% HR 1.363 (95%CI 1.275-1.458). The adjusted probability of being alive with the same or better physical health after 2 years was similar in both systems. However, the VA cohort had a slightly higher adjusted probability of being alive with the same or better mental health score at 2 years (71.8% in the VA vs. 70.1% in MA). Using similar methods, another study by these authors extended the analysis to an approximately five year time frame, with similar results[41]. They found that risk-adjusted mortality rates over an approximately five year period was 26.0% for male VA patients and 28.8% for male Medicare Advantage patients (HR 1.404; 95% CI 1.383–1.426). Among female patients, the unadjusted mortality rates were 20.2% for the VA and 23.4% for the Medicare Advantage program (HR 1.244; 95%CI 1.168–1.324). In a separate analysis, the adjusted rate of 3 year mortality was higher for MA enrollees eligible for Medicaid than in VA enrollees eligible for Medicaid (HR, 1.260 [95% CI, 1.044–1.520])[46].

Harada et al. examined patient satisfaction with outpatient care among VA users compared to non-users in southern California and southern Nevada[45]. VA users were 2 to 8 times more satisfied than VA non-users on 5 of 10 measures of satisfaction. VA users were less satisfied than non-VA users on one measure: the number of days waited for an appointment.

Summary: Of 10 general comparative studies assessing use of preventive services, acute and chronic care for multiple medical acute and chronic medical conditions, changes in broad health status including risk-adjusted morality, and patient satisfaction, each showed superior performance, as measured by greater adherence to accepted processes of care, better health outcomes or improved patient ratings of care, for care delivered in the VA compared with care delivered outside the VA. The studies used data from 1995 to 2004.

CARDIOVASCULAR

We identified 8 studies that assessed quality of care for cardiovascular conditions[24, 34-36, 38, 47-49]. Three studies by Petersen et al. assessed risk-adjusted mortality rates, use of clinically-appropriate coronary angiography, and receipt of effective cardiovascular medications following an acute myocardial infarction among male enrollees in the Medicare fee-for-service program compared to elderly male veterans treated in VA facilities during 1994 and 1995[35, 47]. The authors studied 19,305 male Medicare beneficiaries hospitalized in 1530 nonfederal acute care hospitals for myocardial infarction and 1665 elderly male veterans with myocardial infarction who were treated in 81 VA medical centers. In analyses adjusting for demographic and clinical characteristics, the authors found no difference in mortality for Medicare patients compared with the VA at 30 days (OR 0.94, 95% CI 0.82-1.07) and at one year (OR 0.94, 95% CI 0.84-1.05). Patients in the VA were less likely to receive angiography when clinically needed (43.9 percent vs. 51.0 percent; odds ratio, 0.75; 95% CI, 0.57 to 0.96). After controlling for the availability of on-site cardiac procedures, there was no difference in the rate of angiography[36].

Of the patients who survived their hospitalization, more VA patients than Medicare patients received beta-blockers (49.7 percent vs. 41.6 percent, P<0.001), angiotensin-converting-enzyme inhibitors (44.6 percent vs. 32.5 percent, P<0.001), or aspirin (77.2 percent vs. 68.6 percent, P<0.001) at discharge. Among a subset of patients deemed to be ideal recipients of these medications, VA patients were more likely than Medicare patients to undergo thrombolytic therapy at arrival (OR 1.40 [1.05, 1.74]) or to receive ACE inhibitors (OR 1.67 [1.12, 2.45]) or aspirin (OR 2.32 [1.81, 3.01]) at discharge and equally likely to receive beta-blockers (OR 1.09 [1.03, 1.40]) at discharge[47].

Landrum et al. studied mortality following acute myocardial infarction for elderly male veterans hospitalized in the VA and a matched set of male Medicare beneficiaries treated in non-VA hospitals between 1996 and 1999[34]. The study found that in 1999 there were no significant differences in adjusted 30 day and one year mortality following myocardial infarction between the VA and Medicare. However, in earlier years of the study (1997 and 1998) there were higher adjusted mortality rates in the VA compared to Medicare.

Ritchie et al. compared 10 and 30 day mortality rates and use of cardiac bypass surgery among patients receiving percutaneous coronary angioplasties in a national sample of VA medical centers and a sample of private sector hospitals in the state of Washington[48]. In this study, mortality and bypass surgery rates were largely similar for patients treated in the VA and private sector.

Wright et al. examined mortality rates following an acute myocardial infarction for Medicare-eligible VA-users initially admitted to a VA medical center compared with VA users initially admitted to a Medicare-financed hospital[49]. There were no significant differences in 30 day and 1 year mortality rates for VA users initially admitted to VA medical centers compared to Medicare hospitals.

Another study by Bansal et al. of quality of care for acute myocardial infarction compared use of aspirin, beta-blockers, ace-inhibitors, heparin, and other specified anti-thrombotic agents among patients with an acute myocardial infraction in the Little Rock VA (n=117) compared to patients with acute myocardial infarction in a national sample derived from the National Registry of Myocardial Infarction [24]. The study found higher use of all of these agents in patients at the Little Rock VA compared to those obtaining care elsewhere in Arkansas and to those in the national sample.

Finally, Rehman et al. studied rates of blood pressure control in VA compared to non-VA setting using data from the National Health and Nutrition Examination Survey (NHANES) from 1999 to 2000[38]. The NHANES is a survey of a nationally-representative sample of 5000 persons that is administered by the Centers for Disease Control and Prevention. The survey combines detailed demographic, socioeconomic, nutrition, and health-related questions with a physical examination and laboratory testing by trained medical personnel. The authors found that while blood pressure control to below 140/90 mmHg was comparable among white hypertensive men at VA (55.6%) and non-VA (54.2%) settings (P=.12), blood pressure control was higher among African American hypertensive men at VA (49.4%) compared with non-VA (44.0%) settings (P< 0.01), even after controlling for age, numerous co-morbid conditions, and rural-urban classification.

Summary: Of the 6 studies that assessed cardiovascular outcomes, 5 studies of mortality following an acute myocardial infarction or percutaneous coronary transluminal angioplasty found no clear survival differences between VA and non-VA settings and one study found greater control of blood pressure in the VA. Of the 3 studies that assessed use of processes of care following an acute myocardial infarction, all three found greater rates of evidence-based drug therapy in VA, and one study found lower use of clinically-appropriate angiography in the VA. Of note, all of these cardiovascular studies use data that are between 7 to 18 years old.

DIABETES

We identified 4 studies that focused exclusively on comparing quality of care for diabetes in the VA and outside the VA[31, 39, 50, 51]. Kerr et al. compared clinical performance on 7 diabetes care processes, 3 diabetes intermediate outcomes, and 4 measure of patient satisfaction in 5 VA medical centers and in 8 commercial managed care organizations in matched geographic regions[31]. The study sample included 1285 patients in the VA and 6920 patients in commercial managed care plans. The VA outperformed commercial managed care plans on all measures of care processes. Intermediate outcome of blood pressure control was comparable between the two cohorts; however, the VA cohort had a significantly greater percentage of patients with tight blood sugar and cholesterol control. Patients reported similar overall satisfaction in the two cohorts, though there was significantly greater satisfaction with diabetes care in the VA.

Reiber et al. assessed use of preventive services among veterans with self-reported diabetes using the VA compared with diabetic veterans and non-veterans receiving care outside the VA[39]. The study sample included 535 veterans using VA care, 1848 veterans using non VA care and 9055 nonveterans responding to the 2000 BRFSS. The study found that veterans who used the VA had higher rates of foot exams, diabetes education, and sigmoidoscopy and a lower rate of a1c testing compared to veterans who did not use the VA. There were non-significant differences between these two groups in the receipt of eye exams, blood pressure measurements, cholesterol testing and fecal occult blood testing.

Nelson also examined 2000 BRFSS data and compared use of preventive services among VA enrollees with diabetes compared to persons with diabetes with other sources of insurance coverage[50]. The authors found that persons who received care through the VA were more likely to report taking a diabetes education class than those covered by private insurance The adjusted odds ratio for receipt of diabetes education among persons receiving all of their care through the VA was 3.5 (95% CI 1.6-7.8).

Piette studied satisfaction with care among patient with diabetes treated in 4 VA outpatient clinics compared with patients with diabetes receiving care in a 2 county-funded clinics[51]. The authors found that VA patients were more satisfied than were county patients overall and with 5 of 6 dimensions of their care. These dimensions include access, technical quality, communication, interpersonal care, and quality of outcomes.

Summary: Four studies of the quality of diabetes care demonstrate a performance advantage on some measures for the VA compared with commercial managed care and other non-VA populations.

HOSPITAL AND NURSING HOME CARE

We identified 8 studies that compared the quality of hospital care in the VA with care outside the VA[33, 37, 43, 44, 53, 54, 60, 61].

Polsky et al. examined racial differences in 30 day mortality for patients in VA and non-VA hospitals who were hospitalized for one of six conditions (pneumonia, congestive heart failure, gastrointestinal bleeding, hip fracture, stroke, or acute myocardial infarction)[37]. The data were derived from hospital discharge abstracts from California and Pennsylvania. The study found that among patients less than age 65 years, black patients in VA and non-VA hospitals had similar 30 day mortality rates to whites for gastrointestinal bleeding, hip fracture, and stroke. Among patients 65 years and older, blacks patients in VA and non-VA hospitals had significantly lower odds of 30 day mortality compared to white patients for all conditions except pneumonia. Racial mortality differences for these conditions were similar in VA and non-VA settings.

Weeks et al. compared readmission rates for hospitalized VA enrollees who received care in a VA hospital compared with rates for VA enrollees who were hospitalized in non-VA hospitals[43]. The study included 111,854 patients residing in New York State. Among persons less than age 65, there were no significant differences in 30 day readmission rates for veterans admitted to a VA hospital compared with veterans initially admitted to a non-VA hospital. However, for veterans 65 and older, persons initially admitted to a VA hospital had a significantly higher odds of readmission within 30 days than persons not initially admitted to a VA hospital (OR 2.79, 95%CI 1.4-5.6). In another similar study, Weeks et al. assessed 15 indicators of patient safety for inpatient care provided in VA hospitals compared to care provided outside the VA system[44]. The study found lower risk-adjusted rates of decubitus ulcer, postoperative sepsis, nosocomial infection, postoperative respiratory failure, and postoperative metabolic derangement for VA enrollees hospitalized in VA hospitals compared with rates among VA enrollees treated in hospitals outside the VA. The VA performed worse on one patient safety indicator: mortality rates for low-risk diagnoses. For 9 of the 15 patient safety indicators, there were no significant differences in rates between VA and non-VA hospitals.

Krein et al. assessed the use of central venous catheter bloodstream infection prevention practices in VA and non-VA hospitals using data from survey of a random sample of infection control coordinators in 516 hospitals[33]. The study found that compared with non-VA hospitals, VA hospitals reported greater use of maximal sterile barrier precautions, chlorhexidine gluconate for insertion site antisepsis, and a composite approach using multiple safety practices.

Three similar studies compared hospital mortality rates in a single VA medical center with moratlity rates in different samples of private sector hospitals[53, 54, 61]. Gordon et al. found no significant difference in adjusted mortality rates for the VA medical center compared to a national sample of non-VA hospitals[53]. The actual in-hospital mortality rate was 4.0%, compared with the predicted mortality rate based on the private sector sample of 4.4% (95%CI 4.0% – 4.9%)

Rosenthal also found that risk-adjusted in-hospital mortality was similar in the VA medical center compared with private sector hospitals in the same metropolitan area (OR 1.07 95%CI 0.74-1.54)[60]. Mortality among patients admitted to an intensive care unit was also similar in the VA medical center compared with hospitals in the same metropolitan area[61].

Finally, Berlowitz examined risk-adjusted rates of pressure ulcer development, functional decline, behavioral decline, and mortality in VA nursing homes compared with community nursing homes[54]. Veterans in VA nursing homes were less likely to develop a pressure ulcer (OR 0.62 95%CI 0.47-0.83) but more likely to experience functional decline (OR 1.6 95%CI 1.2-2.1) compared to veterans in community nursing homes. Risk-adjusted mortality and rates of behavioral decline were not different for veterans in VA and community nursing homes.

Summary: Studies of the quality of hospital and nursing home care demonstrate similar risk-adjusted mortality rates in VA facilities compared with non-VA facilities. VA hospitals had somewhat better patient safety outcomes compared with non-VA hospitals. Veterans in VA nursing homes were less likely to develop a pressure ulcer but more likely to experience functional decline compared to veterans in community nursing homes. In addition, the VA had higher use of infection control practices, but greater readmission rates and equivalent mortality rates for racial minorities.

MENTAL HEALTH

We identified 4 studies assessing the quality of mental health care in VA and non-VA settings[26, 55-57]. Busch et al. compared the quality of antidepressant pharmacotherapy in the VA and private sector using identical performance indicators[26]. The authors determined the proportion of patients with a new diagnosis of depression who received a prescription for an antidepressant and remained on antidepressant therapy for the first 84 days following the diagnosis (known as the acute phase of treatment) and for the first 181 days following the diagnosis (known as the maintenance phase of treatment). The VA slightly outperformed the private sector in the prescription of antidepressants during the acute phase of treatment (84.7 compared with 81 percent; $p<0.001$) and during the maintenance phase of treatment (53.9 compared with 50.9 percent; $p<0.001$). The findings persisted when assessed by age and gender.

Leslie et al. compared care for hospitalized patients with schizophrenia in the VA and private sector[55]. Rates of readmission were lower and rates of timely follow-up visits after discharge were higher in the private sector compared to the VA. The VA had better continuity of care, defined as the number of two-month periods in which the patient had two or more outpatient visits in the six months after discharge. In an analysis of the quality of antipsychotic prescribing among patients with schizophrenia, Leslie et al. found that VA patients were more likely to receive a prescription for an antipsychotic and equally likely to be dosed in accordance with accepted clinical guidelines compared to private sector patients with schizophrenia[56].

Finally, Rosenheck examined adherence to 26 treatment guidelines recommended by the Patient Outcomes Research Team (PORT) for patients with schizophrenia[57]. In an analysis of care for patients with schizophrenia in two states in the southeast and Midwest, the study found non-significant differences in adherence to PORT recommendations between VA and non-VA patients for 21 of the 26 measures. Significant differences were found in the following areas: VA outpatients were less likely to receive an antipsychotic medication and to be taking doses outside of the recommended range; VA inpatients were less likely to receive treatment that addressed psychosocial issues than non-VA inpatients; VA outpatients were less likely to participate in work therapy or job training than non-VA outpatients, and both VA inpatients and outpatients were less likely to receive case management services than non-VA patients.

Summary: Studies of the quality of mental health care demonstrate that the quality of antidepressant prescribing is slightly better in VA compared to private sector settings. One study of national data found VA patients with schizophrenia were more likely to receive an antipsychotic medication in the outpatient setting, but a study of data from two states found VA outpatients were less likely to receive an antipsychotic medication and psychosocial services. Among patients discharged after a hospitalization for schizophrenia, readmission and timely outpatient visit follow-up rates after discharge were worse in the VA, but continuity of care in the outpatient setting was better compared to the private sector.

OTHER STUDIES

We classified 4 additional studies into an 'other' category[25, 27, 58, 59].

Barnett et al. compared the use of potentially inappropriate medications among elderly patients in the VA and Medicare managed plans and 10 distinct geographic regions[25]. The authors identified 33 medications that in previously published studies have been generally considered inappropriate when given to the elderly because these medications may pose more risk than benefit. The 33 medications were classified into the following 3 categories: "always avoid", "rarely appropriate" and "some indications'. Compared with Medicare managed care patients, VA patients were less likely to receive any inappropriate medication (21% vs. 29%, P <0.001), and in each classification: always avoid (2% vs. 5%, P <0.001), rarely appropriate (8% vs. 13%, P<0.001), and some indications (15% vs. 17%, P <0.001). The rate of inappropriate drug use was lower in the VA compared with the private sector for both males (21% vs. 24%, P <0.001) and females (28% vs. 32%, P <0.001). Differences were consistent when stratified by age.

Campling et al. examined the survival of Pennsylvania patients diagnosed with lung carcinoma between 1995 and 1999 who were treated in VA medical centers compared to patients treated in other medical centers in the state[27]. The median survival was 6.3 months for VA patients compared with 7.9 months for patients in the rest of the state, and the 5-year overall survival rate was 12% for VA patients compared with 15% for patients in the rest of the state. The Cox model showed a hazard ratio for VA patients compared with non-VA patients of 1.22 (P< 0.001) after adjusting for age, disease stage, and race, meaning that VA patients had a 22% greater odds of dying over the same time period.

Stineman studied functional outcomes following a stroke for patients admitted to 60 VA and 467 non-VA rehabilitation facilities[58]. Across 20 different types of functional impairments, VA patients had significantly better motor outcomes on 8 impairments and worse outcomes for 2 impairments compared to non-VA patients.

Cox et al. compared satisfaction with hearing aid fittings and perceived benefit from hearing aid placement among VA and non-VA patients[59]. VA patients reported greater satisfaction with the fitting of the hearing aid. Using three survey instruments to assess the perceived benefit of using the hearing aid in comparison to unaided hearing, VA patients reported greater benefit on all three instruments. In multivariate analysis of variance adjusting for baseline level of hearing loss, VA had significantly greater benefit from hearing aid placement on a composite measure of all three instruments. When the instruments were examined separately, VA patients reported greater benefit on one instrument but not the other two.

Summary: Elderly VA patients were less likely to be prescribed potentially inappropriate medications than elderly patients in Medicare managed care plans. A study of survival following a diagnosis of lung carcinoma in Pennsylvania found worse survival for VA patients in that state. Stroke patients receiving rehabilitation in VA settings were discharged with better functional outcomes. VA patients had greater satisfaction with hearing aid fittings and somewhat greater self-reported benefit from hearing aid placement.

SUMMARY AND DISCUSSION

LIMITATIONS

PUBLICATION BIAS

Publication bias refers to the lack of publication of studies based on their findings. In its traditional sense, it refers to lack of publication of studies failing to show a statistically significant benefit for an intervention, either because authors feel such results are not newsworthy or because journals are less likely to publish studies that reach null results. In this context, it is not clear whether the specific directionality of a comparison of quality of care between VA and non-VA facilities would lead authors or journal editors to not publish a study. So the potential for publication bias, while always a concern in any systematic review, is not qualitatively the same for this review as in reviews of medical interventions.

However, there is still concern that we identified all published studies of VA care compared to non-VA care. We searched broadly using a literature search strategy designed to identify such articles, but there is never any guarantee that all relevant studies have been found. The consistency of our findings, though, means that any studies that are unpublished would have to be both numerous and have results contrary to the published studies in order to substantively influence our conclusions.

STUDY QUALITY

An important limitation common to systematic reviews is the quality of the original studies. We defined a minimum threshold of design and execution that must have been present for inclusion in our review. Criteria considered included the time frames of the quality measurement in VA and non-VA samples, the similarity of the measures of quality in both samples, the types of measures used, and the statistical methods. Above this threshold, we distinguished between studies based on a global assessment of quality. However, other factors not considered may also have influenced the results of studies in ways we cannot account for.

Ten of the seventeen articles included from the surgical literature were part of the Patient Safety in Surgery Study briefly described previously that used NSQIP methodology to compare care that was provided in the VA setting with that provided in 14 private sector, university hospitals[9, 11-17, 19, 21]. The NSQIP is the first validated, risk adjusted program evaluating outcomes and allowing for measurement of quality of care across surgical settings[62]. However, there are some potential limitations to the Patient Safety in Surgery Study that should be acknowledged. The 14 private sector hospitals in this study may not be generalizable to the private sector at large. Risk adjusted outcomes were assessed in most cases with stepwise logistic regression evaluating the impact of all variables collected on postoperative morbidity and mortality. A potential limitation includes omitted variable bias. For example, risk adjustment models were not able to account for stage of disease in the oncology studies or for indications for surgery in a number of other studies such as those evaluating outcomes after hepatectomy, adrenalectomy, thyroidectomy or parathyroidectomy. The omission of cases may have affected the findings in some studies, as well. For example, in the vascular surgery analyses, endovascular procedures performed outside of the operating room, such as in a radiology suite, were not accounted for. Additionally, in Hall et al's study on thyroidectomies and parathyroidectomies, surgeries performed by otolaryngologists were not captured in the private sector data although they accounted for up to 50% of the operations in the VA[12]. Another limitation was inability to account for specific structural components of the care delivery system. For example, in the Lancaster paper assessing hepatectomy outcomes, the data did not take into account if the hospital had a transplant program, if they were able to perform veno-veno bypass, whether or not specialists in hepatology were on staff and available, ability to perform radiofrequency ablation or the quality of the intensive care units[16]. Finally, morbidity analyses across these studies were based on standard NSQIP assessment of morbidity. Disease and procedure specific outcomes could not be assessed with this data in some instances such as leak rate after pancreatectomy[11], nerve injury after thyroidectomy or parathyroidectomy[12], or disease recurrence after oncologic surgery[11, 19].

An additional limitation is that all but one of the studies was either supported by VA research funding or had VA investigators performing some or all of the work. This may be natural as the VA has more interest than non-VA systems in comparing VA care with non-VA care. However, the possibility of bias must still be kept in mind.

Yet an additional limitation of the non-surgical comparisons is that they are either a narrow set of quality measures applied to a broad set of patients, or a broad set of quality measures applied to a limited sample of patients. In other words, for medical conditions, there is no study that assesses a broad set of quality measures on a national sample of patients. However, the results from the narrow-measures-broad-sample studies and the broad-measures-narrow-sample studies support each other, lessening the likelihood that a broad set of measures applied to a national sample of patients would yield results different from what we report here. Other limitations include lack of comparisons using data collected within the past five years, the use of self-reported data which may be subject to recall error, and the potential for inadequate assessment of clinical risk in studies comparing patient outcomes.

CONCLUSIONS

With the above caveats in mind, we reached the following conclusions for the fifty five articles included in our synthesis. The seventeen surgery articles addressed a variety of conditions and procedures. Primary measures of quality tended to be outcomes measures such as morbidity, mortality, graft survival and occurrence of adverse events. The findings among these seventeen studies were heterogeneous with nine studies reporting no significant difference in quality outcomes, three studies reporting improved quality in the VA compared with the non-VA setting and five reporting improved quality in the non-VA setting. The majority of the surgical studies were based on the Patient Safety in Surgery Study.

Of four general surgery studies, three revealed no significant difference in adjusted postoperative morbidity rates; one found significantly lower rates of postoperative morbidity in the VA setting compared with the private sector. Only 3 of the 4 studies assessed risk adjusted mortality rates; of these two found no significant difference across settings and one found significantly higher risk adjusted rates of postoperative mortality among male patients at the VA compared with the private sector.

Of three solid organ transplant articles, two found no significant difference in patient survival when comparing VA patients with non-VA patients. Additionally, one of these found no significant different in graft survival between these two groups. This study also included a sub-analysis of HRQOL among heart and liver transplant recipients and found no significant different in functional status or mental component scoring, but noted a trend toward lower physical component scores among VA patients after 7 years post-transplant. One study found that VA patients with end-stage renal disease were both less likely to be listed for a kidney transplant and less likely to receive a transplant when listed compared with privately insured patients.

Two of the three vascular surgery studies found significantly lower risk adjusted rates of postoperative morbidity; the final vascular surgery study found no significant difference in morbidity rates. There were no significant differences in risk adjusted mortality rates throughout these three studies.

The studies pertaining to surgical oncology consisted of two that focused on pancreatic cancer and one that focused on breast cancer. One of the pancreatic cancer studies based on the NCDB found no significant difference in postoperative mortality. The other study on pancreatic cancer based on the Patient Safety in Surgery Study found increased risk adjusted postoperative rates of morbidity and mortality. The breast cancer study found no significant difference in risk adjusted postoperative morbidity.

Of the two studies that addressed quality of care related to CABG in VA and non-VA hospitals, one found that, after risk adjustment, VA patients were more likely than non-VA patients to report a problem with patient care. This was based on self-reported data about many aspects of patient care. The second study focused on mortality and found that the odds of death was higher in VA patients relative to private sector patients after accounting for patient level predictors and hospital volume.

In both of the endocrine studies, there were no significant differences in postoperative morbidity or adverse events.

Of 10 general comparative studies assessing use of preventive services, acute and chronic care for multiple medical acute and chronic medical conditions, changes in broad health status including risk-adjusted morality, and patient satisfaction, each showed superior performance, as measured by greater adherence to accepted processes of care, better health outcomes or improved patient ratings of care, for care delivered in the VA compared with care delivered outside the VA. Of the 6 studies that assessed cardiovascular outcomes, 5 studies of mortality following an acute myocardial infarction or percutaneous coronary transluminal angioplasty found no clear survival differences between VA and non-VA settings and one study found greater control of blood pressure in the VA. Of the 3 studies that assessed use of processes of care following an acute myocardial infarction, all three found greater rates of evidence-based drug therapy in VA, but one study found lower use of clinically-appropriate angiography in the VA. Four studies of the quality of diabetes care demonstrate a performance advantage on some measures for the VA compared with commercial managed care and other non-VA populations.

Studies of the quality of hospital and nursing home care demonstrate similar risk-adjusted mortality rates in VA facilities compared with non-VA facilities. VA hospitals had somewhat better patient safety outcomes compared with non-VA hospitals. Veterans in VA nursing homes were less likely to develop a pressure ulcer but more likely to experience functional decline compared to veterans in community nursing homes. In addition, the VA had higher use of infection control practices, but greater readmission rates and equivalent mortality rates across racial groups. Studies of the quality of mental health care demonstrate that the quality of antidepressant prescribing is slightly better in VA compared to private sector settings. One study of national data found VA patients with schizophrenia were more likely to receive an antipsychotic medication in the outpatient setting, but a study of data from two states found VA outpatients were less likely to receive an antipsychotic medication and psychosocial services. Among patients discharged after a hospitalization for schizophrenia, readmission and outpatient visit follow-up rates were worse in the VA, but continuity of care was better compared to the private sector.

Elderly VA patients are less likely to be prescribed potentially inappropriate medications than elderly patients in Medicare managed care plans. A study of survival following a diagnosis of lung carcinoma in Pennsylvania found worse survival for VA patients in that state. Stroke patients receiving rehabilitation in VA settings were discharged with better functional outcomes. VA patients had greater satisfaction with hearing aid fittings and somewhat greater self-reported benefit from hearing aid placement.

Of note, some of the studies compare a narrow band of practice(s), such as vaccinations or a specific type of surgery, across a broader population and other studies compare a wide spectrum of practices in a smaller sample (e.g., Asch et al.)[23]. Moreover, many of the studies are quite dated, with 16 articles using data prior to 2000, and more than likely practices have changed over time inside and outside of the VA.

Overall, the available literature suggests that the care provided in the VA compares favorably to non-VA care systems, albeit with some caveats. Studies that used accepted process of care measures and intermediate outcome measures, such as control of blood pressure or hemoglobin A1c, for quality measurements almost always found VA performed better than non-VA comparison groups. Studies looking at risk-adjusted outcomes generally have found no differences between VA and non-VA care, with some reports of better outcomes in VA and a few reports of worse outcomes in VA, compared to non-VA care. The studies of processes of care are mostly those about medical conditions, while the studies of outcomes are mostly about surgical conditions.

FUTURE RESEARCH

Going forward, further research should be considered to address contemporary comparisons in the quality of care between the VA and the private sector. For example, most of the studies that compared the quality of surgical care in the VA with that in non-VA settings are based on data that is over five years old. The ACS-NSQIP has grown substantially from the original demonstration group of 14 university hospitals in the Patient Safety in Surgery Study to over 180 non-VA hospitals today. The data management for the ACS-NSQIP program has advanced, as well, with more surgical specialties being evaluated and with continually evolving data-fields for collection allowing for more detailed analysis. To further address the quality of care in the VA and non-VA settings, it may be worthwhile to repeat some of these studies using this larger sample; and consideration could be given to merging the VA and ACS NSQIP systems to allow for ongoing comparisons at the institutional and systems level. In areas of medical care, many studies are, as noted with the surgical literature, limited by their age, and newer projects would be worthwhile if benchmarking is considered important. If so, consideration should also be given to determining which healthcare systems the VA should benchmark against (e.g., other managed care organizations, local centers of excellence).

REFERENCE LIST

1. Longman, P., Best Care Anywhere: Why VA Health Care Is Better Than Yours. 2007, Sausalito: PoliPointPress.

2. Ashton, C. M., et al., Hospital use and survival among Veterans Affairs beneficiaries. N Engl J Med, 2003. 349(17): p. 1637-46.

3. Maslin, J. (March 13, 1992) Article 99: Idealism Meets Iodine and Illogic in a Veterans Hospital. New York Times, 99.

4. Canby, V. (December 20, 1989) Born on the Fourth of July: How an All-American Boy Went to War and Lost His Faith. New York Times.

5. Bogdanich, W. (June 29, 2009) Oncologist Defends His Work at a V.A. Hospital. New York Times.

6. Austin, G. L., et al., Comparative analysis of outcome following liver transplantation in US veterans. Am J Transplant, 2004. 4(5): p. 788-95.

7. Bilimoria, K. Y., et al., Quality of pancreatic cancer care at Veterans Administration compared with non-Veterans Administration hospitals. Am J Surg, 2007. 194(5): p. 588-93.

8. Feria, M. I., M. V. Sarrazin and G. E. Rosenthal, Perceptions of care of patients undergoing coronary artery bypass surgery in Veterans Health Administration and private sector hospitals. Am J Med Qual, 2003. 18(6): p. 242-50.

9. Fink, A. S., et al., Comparison of risk-adjusted 30-day postoperative mortality and morbidity in Department of Veterans Affairs hospitals and selected university medical centers: general surgical operations in women. J Am Coll Surg, 2007. 204(6): p. 1127-36.

10. Gill, J. S., et al., Access to kidney transplantation among patients insured by the United States Department of Veterans Affairs. J Am Soc Nephrol, 2007. 18(9): p. 2592-9.

11. Glasgow, R. E., et al., Pancreatic resection in Veterans Affairs and selected university medical centers: results of the patient safety in surgery study. J Am Coll Surg, 2007. 204(6): p. 1252-60.

12. Hall, B. L., et al., Thyroid and parathyroid operations in veterans affairs and selected university medical centers: results of the patient safety in surgery study. J Am Coll Surg, 2007. 204(6): p. 1222-34.

13. Henderson, W. G., et al., Comparison of risk-adjusted 30-day postoperative mortality and morbidity in Department of Veterans Affairs hospitals and selected university medical centers: general surgical operations in men. J Am Coll Surg, 2007. 204(6): p. 1103-14.

14. Hutter, M. M., et al., Comparison of risk-adjusted 30-day postoperative mortality and morbidity in Department of Veterans Affairs hospitals and selected university medical centers: vascular surgical operations in men. J Am Coll Surg, 2007. 204(6): p. 1115-26.

15. Johnson, R. G., et al., Comparison of risk-adjusted 30-day postoperative mortality and morbidity in Department of Veterans Affairs hospitals and selected university medical centers: vascular surgical operations in women. J Am Coll Surg, 2007. 204(6): p. 1137-46.

16. Lancaster, R. T., et al., Liver resection in veterans affairs and selected university medical centers: results of the patient safety in surgery study. J Am Coll Surg, 2007. 204(6): p. 1242-51.

17. Lautz, D. B., et al., Bariatric operations in Veterans Affairs and selected university medical centers: results of the patient safety in surgery study. J Am Coll Surg, 2007. 204(6): p. 1261-72.

18. Moore, D., et al., Survival and quality of life after organ transplantation in veterans and nonveterans. Am J Surg, 2003. 186(5): p. 476-80.

19. Neumayer, L., et al., Breast cancer surgery in Veterans Affairs and selected university medical centers: results of the patient safety in surgery study. J Am Coll Surg, 2007. 204(6): p. 1235-41.

20. Rosenthal, G. E., M. Vaughan Sarrazin and E. L. Hannan, In-hospital mortality following coronary artery bypass graft surgery in Veterans Health Administration and private sector hospitals. Med Care, 2003. 41(4): p. 522-35.

21. Turrentine, F. E., et al., Adrenalectomy in Veterans Affairs and selected university medical centers: results of the patient safety in surgery study. J Am Coll Surg, 2007. 204(6): p. 1273-83.

22. Weiss, J. S., et al., Safety of carotid endarterectomy in a high-risk population: lessons from the VA and Connecticut. J Am Coll Surg, 2006. 203(3): p. 277-82.

23. Asch, S. M., et al., Comparison of quality of care for patients in the Veterans Health Administration and patients in a national sample. Ann Intern Med, 2004. 141(12): p. 938-45.

24. Bansal, D., et al., Trends in the care of patients with acute myocardial infarction at a university-affiliated Veterans Affairs Medical Center. J Cardiovasc Pharmacol Ther, 2005. 10(1): p. 39-44.

25. Barnett, M. J., et al., Comparison of rates of potentially inappropriate medication use according to the Zhan criteria for VA versus private sector medicare HMOs. J Manag Care Pharm, 2006. 12(5): p. 362-70.

26. Busch, S. H., D. L. Leslie and R. A. Rosenheck, Comparing the quality of antidepressant pharmacotherapy in the Department of Veterans Affairs and the private sector. Psychiatr Serv, 2004. 55(12): p. 1386-91.

27. Campling, B. G., et al., A population-based study of lung carcinoma in Pennsylvania: comparison of Veterans Administration and civilian populations. Cancer, 2005. 104(4): p. 833-40.

28. Chi, R. C., G. E. Reiber and K. M. Neuzil, Influenza and pneumococcal vaccination in older veterans: results from the behavioral risk factor surveillance system. J Am Geriatr Soc, 2006. 54(2): p. 217-23.

29. Jha, A. K., et al., Effect of the transformation of the Veterans Affairs Health Care System on the quality of care. N Engl J Med, 2003. 348(22): p. 2218-27.

30. Jha, A. K., S. M. Wright and J. B. Perlin, Performance measures, vaccinations, and pneumonia rates among high-risk patients in Veterans Administration health care. Am J Public Health, 2007. 97(12): p. 2167-72.

31. Kerr, E. A., et al., Diabetes care quality in the Veterans Affairs Health Care System and commercial managed care: the TRIAD study. Ann Intern Med, 2004. 141(4): p. 272-81.

32. Keyhani, S., et al., Use of preventive care by elderly male veterans receiving care through the Veterans Health Administration, Medicare fee-for-service, and Medicare HMO plans. Am J Public Health, 2007. 97(12): p. 2179-85.

33. Krein, S. L., et al., Use of central venous catheter-related bloodstream infection prevention practices by US hospitals. Mayo Clin Proc, 2007. 82(6): p. 672-8.

34. Landrum, M. B., et al., Care following acute myocardial infarction in the Veterans Administration Medical Centers: a comparison with Medicare. Health Serv Res, 2004. 39(6 Pt 1): p. 1773-92.

35. Petersen, L. A., et al., Outcome of myocardial infarction in Veterans Health Administration patients as compared with medicare patients. N Engl J Med, 2000. 343(26): p. 1934-41.

36. Petersen, L. A., et al., Regionalization and the underuse of angiography in the Veterans Affairs Health Care System as compared with a fee-for-service system. N Engl J Med, 2003. 348(22): p. 2209-17.

37. Polsky, D., et al., Is lower 30-day mortality posthospital admission among blacks unique to the Veterans Affairs health care system? Med Care, 2007. 45(11): p. 1083-9.

38. Rehman, S. U., et al., Ethnic differences in blood pressure control among men at Veterans Affairs clinics and other health care sites. Arch Intern Med, 2005. 165(9): p. 1041-7.

39. Reiber, G. E., et al., Diabetes in nonveterans, veterans, and veterans receiving Department of Veterans Affairs health care. Diabetes Care, 2004. 27 Suppl 2: p. B3-9.

40. Ross, J. S., et al., Use of recommended ambulatory care services: is the Veterans Affairs quality gap narrowing? Arch Intern Med, 2008. 168(9): p. 950-8.

41. Selim, A. J., et al., Risk-adjusted mortality as an indicator of outcomes: comparison of the Medicare Advantage Program with the Veterans' Health Administration. Med Care, 2006. 44(4): p. 359-65.

42. Selim, A. J., et al., Change in health status and mortality as indicators of outcomes: comparison between the Medicare Advantage Program and the Veterans Health Administration. Qual Life Res, 2007. 16(7): p. 1179-91.

43. Weeks, W. B., et al., Comparing the characteristics, utilization, efficiency, and outcomes of VA and non-VA inpatient care provided to VA enrollees: a case study in New York. Med Care, 2008. 46(8): p. 863-71.

44. Weeks, W. B., et al., Comparing measures of patient safety for inpatient care provided to veterans within and outside the VA system in New York. Qual Saf Health Care, 2008. 17(1): p. 58-64.

45. Harada, N. D., V. M. Villa and R. Andersen, Satisfaction with VA and non-VA outpatient care among veterans. Am J Med Qual, 2002. 17(4): p. 155-64.

46. Selim, A. J., et al., Differences in risk-adjusted mortality between medicaid-eligible patients enrolled in medicare advantage plans and those enrolled in the veterans health administration. J Ambul Care Manage, 2009. 32(3): p. 232-40.

47. Petersen, L. A., et al., Comparison of use of medications after acute myocardial infarction in the Veterans Health Administration and Medicare. Circulation, 2001. 104(24): p. 2898-904.

48. Ritchie, J. L., et al., A comparison of percutaneous transluminal coronary angioplasty in the Department of Veterans Affairs and in the private sector in the State of Washington. Am J Cardiol, 1998. 81(9): p. 1094-9.

49. Wright, S. M., et al., Increasing use of Medicare services by veterans with acute myocardial infarction. Med Care, 1999. 37(6): p. 529-37.

50. Nelson, K. M., et al., The association between health insurance coverage and diabetes care; data from the 2000 Behavioral Risk Factor Surveillance System. Health Serv Res, 2005. 40(2): p. 361-72.

51. Piette, J. D., Satisfaction with care among patients with diabetes in two public health care systems. Med Care, 1999. 37(6): p. 538-46.

52. Weeks, W. B., et al., Veterans Health Administration and Medicare outpatient health care utilization by older rural and urban New England veterans. J Rural Health, 2005. 21(2): p. 167-71.

53. Gordon, H. S., et al., Using severity-adjusted mortality to compare performance in a Veterans Affairs hospital and in private-sector hospitals. Am J Med Qual, 2000. 15(5): p. 207-11.

54. Berlowitz, D. R., et al., Purchasing or providing nursing home care: can quality of care data provide guidance. J Am Geriatr Soc, 2005. 53(4): p. 603-8.

55. Leslie, D. L. and R. A. Rosenheck, Comparing quality of mental health care for public-sector and privately insured populations. Psychiatr Serv, 2000. 51(5): p. 650-5.

56. Leslie, D. L. and R. A. Rosenheck, Benchmarking the quality of schizophrenia pharmacotherapy: a comparison of the Department of Veterans Affairs and the private sector. J Ment Health Policy Econ, 2003. 6(3): p. 113-21.

57. Rosenheck, R. A., et al., Benchmarking treatment of schizophrenia: a comparison of service delivery by the national government and by state and local providers. J Nerv Ment Dis, 2000. 188(4): p. 209-16.

58. Stineman, M. G., et al., Inpatient rehabilitation after stroke: a comparison of lengths of stay and outcomes in the Veterans Affairs and non-Veterans Affairs health care system. Med Care, 2001. 39(2): p. 123-37.

59. Cox, R. M., G. C. Alexander and G. A. Gray, Hearing aid patients in private practice and public health (Veterans Affairs) clinics: are they different? Ear Hear, 2005. 26(6): p. 513-28.

60. Rosenthal, G. E., et al., Mortality and length of stay in a veterans affairs hospital and private sector hospitals serving a common market. J Gen Intern Med, 2003. 18(8): p. 601-8.

61. Kaboli, P. J., et al., Length of stay as a source of bias in comparing performance in VA and private sector facilities: lessons learned from a regional evaluation of intensive care outcomes. Med Care, 2001. 39(9): p. 1014-24.

62. Khuri, S. F., et al., The Department of Veterans Affairs' NSQIP: the first national, validated, outcome-based, risk-adjusted, and peer-controlled program for the measurement and enhancement of the quality of surgical care. National VA Surgical Quality Improvement Program. Ann Surg, 1998. 228(4): p. 491-5.

APPENDICES

APPENDIX 1. EVIDENCE TABLE OF SURGICAL STUDIES

Author; Year	Category	VA Sample			Non-VA Sample			Conditions	Outcomes	Primary Findings	Final Grade
		Data Level	Sample Size	Years Collected	Data Level	Sample Size	Years Collected				
Austin, G.L., et al.; 2004[6]	Solid Organ Transplantation	Single ctr	149	1991-2000	Single med ctr	285	1991-2000	Other Surgical	mortality at 1,3,5 years	VA patients had increased mortality rates as assessed by Kaplan-Meier curves. However after adjusting for gender, donor age, recipient age, etiology of liver disease and MELD score, hospital status was not a significant predictor of mortality RR 1.15 (95% CI 0.94-1.43)	A
Bilimoria, K.Y., et al.; 2007[7]	Oncology	Nat'l	513	1985-2004	Nat'l	12,756/ 18,299	1985-2004	General surgical, Surgical Oncology	60 day and 3 year mortality	Unadjusted and adjusted mortality rates at 60days and 3 years were comparable between VA, academic and community hospital settings for resection of stage I and II pancreatic cancer.	B
Feria, M.I., et al.; 2003[8]	Cardiac	Nat'l	808	1995-1998	Mult ctrs	18,299	1996-1998	IHD, Cardiothoracic	perceptions of various dimensions of care	VA patients were more likely than non-VA patients to note a problem with patient care; when analysis limited to teaching hospital settings, VA patients remained more likely to note a problem with care in 5 dimensions.	B

Comparison of Quality of Care in VA and Non-VA Settings

Author; Year	Category	VA Sample			Non-VA Sample			Conditions	Outcomes	Primary Findings	Final Grade
		Data Level	Sample Size	Years Collected	Data Level	Sample Size	Years Collected				
Fink, A.S., et al.; 2007[9]	General	Nat'l	5157	2001-2004	Mult. Ctrs	27467	2001-2004	General surgical	30 day postoperative morbidity and mortality	Risk adjusted mortality rates are comparable between PS and VA patients, although setting of care did not enter the mortality regression model. Risk adjusted morbidity was higher in the PS compared with the VA OR 0.8 (CI 0.71-0.90)	B
Gill, J.S., et al.; 2007[10]	Solid Organ Transplantation	Nat'l	7395	1995-2004	Nat'l	144651/ 357345	1995-2004	Other surgical	time to treatment	Both VA-insured and Medicare/Medicaid-insured patients were approximately 35% less likely to receive transplants than patients with private insurance (hazard ratio [HR] 0.65; 95% CI 0.60 to 0.70; P_ 0.0001). Most of this difference was explained by the fact that VA patients were less likely to be placed on the wait-list (HR 0.71; 95% CI 0.67 to 0.76), but even listed VA patients received transplants less frequently (HR 0.89; 95% CI 0.82 to 0.96).	A
Glasgow, R.E., et al.; 2007[11]	Oncology	Nat'l	377	2001-2004	Mult. Ctrs	692	2001-2004	Other surgical	postoperative outcomes (primarily morbidity and mortality)	Adjusting for case mix differences, postoperative morbidity and mortality rates for pancreatectomy were higher in the VA compared with the PS (OR 1.581, 95% CI 1.084-2.307 and 2.533 95% CI 1.020– 6.290 respectively).	A/B

Comparison of Quality of Care in VA and Non-VA Settings

Author, Year	VA Sample				Non-VA Sample				Conditions	Outcomes	Primary Findings	Final Grade
	Category	Data Level	Sample Size	Years Collected	Data Level	Sample Size	Years Collected					
Hall, B.L., et al.; 2007[12]	Endocrine	Nat'l	2814	2001-2004	Mult. Ctrs	357345	2001-2004		General surgical, head and neck	30 day morbidity and mortality; specific adverse event rates, LOS	Overall 30day morbidity and mortality do not differ significantly in the VA vs PS in risk adjusted model. Mortality event rate is too low to accurately evaluate, odds ratio for morbidity associated with VA care is 1.25 (95% CI 0.87-1.78)	B
Henderson, W.G., et al.; 2007[13]	General	Nat'l	9409818	2001-2004	Mult. Ctrs	18399	2001-2004		General surgical	30 day postoperative morbidity and mortality	After risk adjustment for patient comorbidities and severity of illness, the odds of mortality at 30days were higher in the VA compared with the PS (OR 1.23, 95% CI). There was no significant difference in morbidity at 30days among the sites.	A/B
Hutter, M.M., et al.; 2007[14]	Vascular	Nat'l	5174	2001-2004	Mult. Ctrs	30058	2001-2004		Vascular	30 day postoperative morbidity and mortality	Risk adjusted mortality was comparable among the two groups, although hospital site/type did not enter the stepwise regression model. Accounting for comorbidities and severity of illness, postoperative morbidity rates were lower in the VA population, OR 0.84 (95% CI 0.78-0.92)	A/B

Comparison of Quality of Care in VA and Non-VA Settings

Author; Year	Category	VA Sample				Non-VA Sample			Conditions	Outcomes	Primary Findings	Final Grade
		Data Level	Sample Size	Years Collected	Data Level	Sample Size	Years Collected					
Johnson, R.G., et al.; 2007[15]	Vascular	Nat'l	458	2001-2004	Mult. Ctrs	3535	2001-2004	Vascular	30 day postoperative morbidity and mortality	After risk adjustment, no significant difference in 30 day mortality rates among VA and PS female vascular patients. After adjusting for severity of illness, 30 day complication/morbidity rates were significantly lower in the VA compared with the PS (OR 0.60, 95% CI 0.44-0.81)	B
Lancaster, R.T., et al.; 2007[16]	General	Nat'l	237	2001-2004	Mult. Ctrs	783	2001-2004	General surgical	post-operative morbidity and mortality at 30 days; also evaluated LOS, need for re-operation and occurrence of 18 specific postoperative events	Risk adjusted outcomes suggest that 30day post-operative morbidity and mortality rates in the VA compared with the PS for hepatic resections do not vary significantly. (after risk adjustment, morbidity rates and mortality were comparable in VA and PS. Comparing Morbidity of VA w/PS OR was 0.94 (95% CI 0.62-1.42) and Mortality OR was 1.623 (95% CI 0.61-4.32))	A/B

Comparison of Quality of Care in VA and Non-VA Settings

Author; Year	Category	VA Sample			Non-VA Sample			Conditions	Outcomes	Primary Findings	Final Grade
		Data Level	Sample Size	Years Collected	Data Level	Sample Size	Years Collected				
Lautz, D.B., et al.; 2007[17]	General	Nat'l	374	2001-2004	Mult. Ctrs	2064	2001-2004	Other surgical	30 day postoperative outcomes: morbidity (overall, specific adverse events, # complications), mortality, LOS	No significant difference in postop morbidity or mortality among women in the VA versus non-VA settings (16.07 vs 12.02 % p =0.21 and 0.89 vs 0.42%, p=0.47). Unadjusted and adjusted morbidity rates were higher among men treated at the VA versus non-VA (OR 2.77, 95% CI 1.78-4.31 unadjusted and OR 2.29, 95% CI 1.28-4.10 adjusted). Unadjusted mortality rates significantly higher among men treated at VA versus non-VA((1.91% vs 0.25% p=0.03).	A/B
Moore, D., et al.; 2003[18]	Solid Organ Transplantation	Single ctr	380	1990-2002	Single med ctr	1429	1990-2002	Other surgical	graft survival; patient survival, Karnofsky score, SF36	No significant difference in graft or patient survival in liver, heart, or kidney between veteran and nonveteran patients, and survival statistics were consistent with recently published national data	A
Neumayer, L., et al.; 2007[19]	Oncology	Nat'l	644	2001-2004	Mult. Ctrs	3179	2001-2004	General surgical	30day postoperative morbidity and mortality, LOS	After adjusting for comorbidities and preoperative factors, there was no significant difference in 30day morbidity or mortality in female patients at the VA compared with the PS (OR 1.404, 95% CI 0.894-2.204).	B

Comparison of Quality of Care in VA and Non-VA Settings

Author; Year	Category	VA Sample Data Level	VA Sample Size	VA Years Collected	Non-VA Data Level	Non-VA Sample Size	Non-VA Years Collected	Conditions	Outcomes	Primary Findings	Final Grade
Rosenthal, G.E., et al.; 2003[20]	Cardiac	Nat'l	19266	1993-1996	Lrg geo area	44247/ 9696	1993-1996	Cardio-thoracic	in hospital mortality	Adjusting for patient-level predictors and volume, the odds of death was higher in VA patients, relative to private sector patients (OR, 1.34; 95% CI, 1.11-1.63; P <0.001).	A
Turrentine F.E., et al.; 2007[21]	Endocrine	Nat'l	178	2001-2004	Mult. Ctrs	371	2001-2004	Other surgical	30 day morbidity and mortality	Unadjusted morbidity and mortality rates were higher in VA compared with PS (16.3% vs 6.7%, p=0.003 and 2.8% vs. 0.4%, p=0.0074). Mortality event rate was too low for adjustment. Adjusting for comorbidities, the 30day postoperative morbidity ratio in the VA versus the PS was no longer significant (adjusted OR1.33, 95%CI 0.49-3.6 compared with unadjusted OR 2.75, 95% CI: 1.55-4.91).	B
Weiss, J.S., et al.; 2006[22]	Vascular	One VISN	140	1997-2002	Lrg geo	6949	1997-2002	Vascular	perioperative mortality, stroke and cardiac complications	After risk adjustment, having surgery at the VA was not a significant predictor of death (OR 2.98, 95% CI 0.51-17.6), stroke (OR .95, 95% CI 0.3-3.4) or cardiac complications(OR 1.07 95% CI 0.37-3.1)	B

APPENDIX 2. EVIDENCE TABLE OF MEDICAL AND NON-SURGICAL STUDIES

Author; Year	Category	VA Sample			Non-VA Sample			Conditions	Outcomes	Primary Findings	Final Grade
		Data Level	Sample Size	Years Collected	Data Level	Sample Size	Years Collected				
Asch, S.M., et al.; 2004[23]	General, mult conditions	Mult. VISNs	596	1997-1999	Nat'l	992	1996-2000	CHF, DM, IHD, HTN, Pulmonary Disease, Preventive Care, Cancer, Osteoarthritis, Depression, TIA/Stroke	adherence to 348 indicators targeting 26 conditions	VA scored better on adjusted overall quality 67% vs 51%; chronic disease care (72 vs 59) and preventive care (64 vs 44), but not acute care.	A
Bansal, D., et al.; 2005[24]	Cardiovascular	Single ctr	92/117	2002	Nat'l	not described	2002	IHD	use of aspirin, betablockers, aceinhibitors, heparin, gp2a3b inhibitors among pts with MI	Use of all these agents were higher in the Little Rock VA compared to the rest of Arkansas and the entire US	B
Barnett, M.J., et al.; 2006[25]	Other	Nat'l	123633	2002-2003	Nat'l	157517	2000-2001	Other safety	use of potentially inappropriate medications among the elderly	Compared with private sector patients, VA patients were less likely to receive any inappropriate medication (21% vs. 29%, P <0.001), and in each classifcation: always avoid (2% vs. 5%, P <0.001), rarely appropriate (8% vs. 13%, P<0.001), and some indications (15% vs. 17%, P <0.001).	B

Comparison of Quality of Care in VA and Non-VA Settings

| Author; Year | Category | VA Sample | | | Non-VA Sample | | | Conditions | Outcomes | Primary Findings | Final Grade |
		Data Level	Sample Size	Years Collected	Data Level	Sample Size	Years Collected				
Berlowitz, D.R., et al.; 2005[54]	Hospital and nursing home care	One VISN	3802/961	1997-1999	Lrg geo area	52986/ 142452	1997-1999	Other medical/ nonsurgical condition	Risk-adjusted rates of pressure ulcer development, functional decline, behavioral decline, and mortality.	Veterans in VA nursing homes were significantly (P<.05) less likely to develop a pressure ulcer (odds ratio (OR)=0.63) but more likely to experience functional decline (OR=1.6) than veterans in community nursing homes. Veterans in VA nursing homes were also less likely to die but more likely to experience behavioral decline, but these differences did not achieve statistical significance after risk adjustment.	A
Busch, S.H., et al.; 2004[26]	Mental health care	Nat'l	27713	2000-2001	Nat'l	4852	2000-2001	Depression	Receipt of 84, 140, and 181 of antidepressant therapy among patients with initial diagnosis of depression	The VA slightly outperformed the private sector in the prescription of antidepressants during the acute phase of treatment, the first 84 days (84.7 compared with 81 percent) and during the maintenance phase of treatment, the first 181 days (53.9 compared with 50.9 percent). The findings persisted after adjustment for age and sex but lost significance after adjustment for comorbid conditions.	A

Comparison of Quality of Care in VA and Non-VA Settings

Author, Year	Category	VA Sample			Non-VA Sample			Conditions	Outcomes	Primary Findings	Final Grade
		Data Level	Sample Size	Years Collected	Data Level	Sample Size	Years Collected				
Campling, B.G., et al.; 2005[27]	Other	One VISN	862	1995-1999	Lrg geo	27936	1995-1999	Cancer	survival following diagnosis of lung cancer	The median survival was 6.3 months for VA patients compared with 7.9 months for patients in the rest of the state, and the 5-year overall survival rate was 12% for VA patients compared with 15% for patients in the rest of the state. The Cox model showed a hazard ratio for VA patients compared with non-VA patients of 1.22 (P_ 0.001) after adjusting for age, disease stage, and race.	B
Chi, R.C., et al.; 2006[28]	General, prevention	Nat'l	3265	2003	Nat'l	10677/ 40331	2003	Preventive Care	Influenza and pneumococcal vaccination	Among veterans, Influenza and vccinatin rates highers for VA users compared to non-users. For veterans, VA care was independently associated with influenza vaccination (adjusted OR 1.8; 95%CI 1-5-2.2) and pneumococcal vaccionation (adjusted OR 2.4; 95%CI 2.0-2.9).	A
Cox, R.M., et al.; 2005[59]	Other	Mult VISNs	151	2000-2003	Mult ctrs	79	2000-2003	Other medical/ nonsurgical condition	satisfaction with hearing aid fitting	Three weeks after the fitting, VA patients reported more satisfaction with their hearing aids. On some measures VA patients reported more benefit, but different measures of benefit did not give completely consistent results.	B

Comparison of Quality of Care in VA and Non-VA Settings

Author; Year	Category	VA Sample				Non-VA Sample			Conditions	Outcomes	Primary Findings	Final Grade
		Data Level	Sample Size	Years Collected	Data Level	Sample Size	Years Collected					
Gordon, H.S., et al.; 2000[53]	Hospital and nursing home care	Single ctr	5016	1993	Nat'l	850000	1991	Other medical/ nonsurgical condition	hospital mortality	Adjusted death rates were similar in the VA and a private sector sample	B
Harada, N.D., et al.; 2002[45]	General, patient satisfaction	One VISN	1262/840 dual	2000	Lrg geo areao	550	2000	Other medical/ nonsurgical condition	patient satisfaction with outpatient care	VA users were 2-8 times more satisfied than va non-users on 5 of 10 measures of satisfaction. VA users were less satified than non-VA users on one measure – number of days waited for an appointment.	B
Jha, A.K, et al.; 2003[29]	General, mult conditions	Nat'l	48505-84503	1994-2000	Nat'l	diff. to ascertain	1997-2001	CHF, DM, IHD, Preventive care	3 preventive measures, 3 diabetes measures, 5 ami measures, 2 chf measures	The VA outperformed the Medicare fee-for-service program on all 11 similar indicators from 1997 to 1999 and of 12 of 13 indicators in 2000.	A
Jha, A.K, et al.; 2007[30]	General, prevention	Nat'l	48505-84503	1994-2000	Nat'l	diff. to ascertain	1997-2001	Preventive Care	3 preventive measures, 3 diabetes measures, 5 ami measures, 2 chf measures	The VA outperformed the Medicare fee-for-service program on all 11 similar indicators from 1997 to 1999 and of 12 of 13 indicators in 2000.	A
Kaboli, P.J., et al.; 2001[61]	Hospital and nursing home care	Single ctr	1142	1994-1995	Mult ctrs	51249	1994-1995	Other medical/ nonsurgical condition	risk adjusted mortality	Using logistic regression to adjust for severity, the odds of death was similar in VA patients, relative to private sector patients (OR 1.16, 95% CI 0.93-1.44; P = 0.18). Using proportional hazards regression and censoring patients at hospital discharge, the risk for death was lower in VA patients (hazard ratio 0.70; 95% CI 0.59-0.82; P <0.001).	B

Comparison of Quality of Care in VA and Non-VA Settings

| Author; Year | Category | VA Sample | | | Non-VA Sample | | | Conditions | Outcomes | Primary Findings | Final Grade |
		Data Level	Sample Size	Years Collected	Data Level	Sample Size	Years Collected				
Kerr, E.A., et al.; 2004[31]	Diabetes	Mult. VISNs	1285	2000-2001	Mult. Ctrs	6616	2001-2002	DM	Process of care measures of quality as derived from the Diabetes Quality Improvement, Project accountability and measurement set, Intermediate outcomes, Patient satisfaction with care	After adjustment, VA significantly outperformed mgd care on all process of care measures. Intermediate outcome of blood pressure control was comparable between the two cohorts, however the VA cohort had significantly greater percentage of patients tight HgbA1C and LDL control. Patients reported similar overall satisfaction in the two cohorts, though there was significantly greater satisfaction with diabetes care in the VA.	A
Keyhani, S., et al.; 2007[32]	General, prevention	Nat'l	171/ 1009/145	2000-2003	Nat'l	3552/576	2000-2003	Preventive Care	self-reported use of influenza vaccination, pneumonia vaccianation, serum cholesterol screening	Veterans receiving care through VA reported 10% greater use of influenza vaccination (P<.05), 14% greater use of pneumococcal vaccination (P<.01), And a nonsignificant 6% greater use of serum cholesterol screening (P=.1), than did veterans receiving care through Medicare HMOs. Veterans receiving care through Medicare FFS reported less use of all 4 preventive measures (P<.01) than did veterans receiving care through Medicare HMOs.	B

Comparison of Quality of Care in VA and Non-VA Settings

Author; Year	Category	VA Sample				Non-VA Sample				Conditions	Outcomes	Primary Findings	Final Grade
		Data Level	Sample Size	Years Collected		Data Level	Sample Size	Years Collected					
Krein, S.L., et al.; 2007[33]	Hospital and nursing home care	Nat'l	95 hospitals	2005		Nat'l	421 hospitals	2005		Other medical/ nonsurgical condition	regular use of specific prevention modalities (maximum sterile barrier precautions, use of chlorhexadine gluconate for insertion site and antimicrobial CV catheters, routine change of catheters, use of antimicrobial impreganated dressing); also a composite measure of max sterile barrier, chlorhexadine and avoidance of routine changes.	Adjusted findings revealed that VA hospitals were significantly more likely to use chlorhexadine gluconate (OR 4.8, 95%CI 1.6-15.0) and/or to use a composite approach (OR 2.1, 95%CI 1.0-4.2) as compared with non-VA hospitals.	B
Landrum, M.B., et al.; 2004[34]	Cardio-vascular	Nat'l	15259/ 13129	1996-1999		Nat'l	447445/ 384470	1996-1999		IHD	mortality (30 day and one year)	VA pts had significantly higher one year mortality rates across all years studied; 30day mortality rates were higher in VA in 1997 however 30day mortality rates decreased overtime and were comparable between the two sites by 1999.	B

Comparison of Quality of Care in VA and Non-VA Settings

Author, Year	Category	VA Sample			Non-VA Sample			Conditions	Outcomes	Primary Findings	Final Grade
		Data Level	Sample Size	Years Collected	Data Level	Sample Size	Years Collected				
Leslie, D.L., et al.; 2000[55]	Mental health	Nat'l	181132	1993-1997	Nat'l	12163	1993-1995	Depression, Psychosis/ schizo- phrenia, other medical/ nonsurgical condition	Readmission rates and outpatient follow-up care following hospitalization for a psychiatric or substance abuse disorder	This study found that, overall, private-sector mental health inpatients had shorter lengths of stay, more days to the next inpatient readmission, and lower readmission rates within 14, 30, or 180 days of discharge compared with VA mental health inpatients. Although VA patients had higher continuity-of-care scores, moderately higher proportions of private-sector patients had an outpatient visit within 30 and 180 days after discharge. Private-sector patients also had fewer days to the first outpatient visit and more outpatient visits in the six months after discharge.	B
Leslie, D.L., et al.; 2003[56]	Mental health	Nat'l	2636	2000	Nat'l	1318	2000	Psychosis/ schizo- phrenia	adherence to treatment guidelines for antipsychotic prescribing	Patients in the VA and private sector were equally likely to receive an antipsychotic regimen that complied with PORT guidelines.	B
Nelson, K.M., et al.; 2005[50]	Diabetes	Nat'l	254/281	2000	Nat'l	10632	2000	DM	They studied five self-reported measures of diabetes self-management and preventive care practices	Persons who received care through the VA were more likely to report taking a diabetes education class and HbA1c testing than those covered by private insurance.	B

Comparison of Quality of Care in VA and Non-VA Settings

Author; Year	Category	VA Sample Data Level	VA Sample Size	VA Years Collected	Non-VA Data Level	Non-VA Sample Size	Non-VA Years Collected	Conditions	Outcomes	Primary Findings	Final Grade
Petersen, L.A., et al.; 2000[35]	Cardiovascular	Nat'l	2486/ 13310	1994-1995	Nat'l	29249/ 41754	1994-1995	IHD	comparison of coexisting conditions, severity of AMI and mortality at 30days & one year	Adjusted rates of mortality at 30days and one year were not significantly different among VA and Medicare patients after AMI (OR 0.94, 95% CI 0.82-1.07 and OR 0.94, 95% CI 0.84-1.05 respectively).	B
Petersen, L.A., et al.; 2001[47]	Cardiovascular	Nat'l	2486	1994-1995	Nat'l	29249	1994-1995	IHD	use of thrombolytics, β-blockers, ACE inhibitors, or aspirin among ideal candidates following an acute myocardial infarction	Ideal VA candidates were more likely to undergo thrombolytic therapy at arrival (OR [VA relative to Medicare] 1.40 [1.05, 1.74]) or to receive ACE inhibitors (OR 1.67 [1.12, 2.45]) or aspirin (OR 2.32 [1.81, 3.01]) at discharge and equally likely to receive β-blockers (OR 1.09 [1.03, 1.40]) at discharge.	A
Petersen, L.A., et al.; 2003[36]	Cardiovascular	Nat'l	1665/ 2486	1994-1995	Nat'l	19305/ 29249	1994-1995	IHD	use of angiography (appropriate use) and mortality	After accounting for patient characteristics and need for angiography, VA pts were significantly less likely to receive angiography (43.9 vs 51%, OR 0.75, 95% CI 0.57-0.96). After accounting for hospital and capability of cardiac interventions, underuse of angiography and mortality did not differ significantly between patient groups.	A
Piette, J.D.; 1999[51]	Diabetes	Mult ctrs	310	1996-1997	Mults ctrs	228	1996-1997	DM	Six dimensions of patient satisfaction	VA patients were more satisfied than were county patients overall and with 5 of 6 dimensions of their care.	B

Comparison of Quality of Care in VA and Non-VA Settings

| Author; Year | Category | VA Sample | | | Non-VA Sample | | | Conditions | Outcomes | Primary Findings | Final Grade |
		Data Level	Sample Size	Years Collected	Data Level	Sample Size	Years Collected				
Polsky, D., et al.; 2007[37]	Hospital and nursing home care	Nat'l	369155/ 427367	1995-2001	Lrg geo	1509891/ 3861953	1995-2001	CHF, IHD, Pulmonary Disease, TIA/Stroke	30 day mortality (for white and black males after hospital admission for any of the above conditions)	After risk adjustment, racial (black vs white) differences in 30 day mortality rates after admission for 6 medical conditions were similar among VA and non-VA care settings.	B
Rehman, S.U., et al.; 2005[38]	Cardio-vascular	One VISN	12366	2001-2003	Lrg geo	7734	2001-2003	HTN	control of blood pressure below 140/90	Blood pressure control to below 140/90 mmHg was comparable among white hypertensive men at VA (55.6%) and non-VA (54.2%) settings (P=.12). In contrast, BP control was higher among African American hypertensive men at VA (49.4%) compared with non-VA (44.0%) settings (P_.01), even after controlling for age, numerous comorbid conditions, and rural/urban classification. Being in a non-VA site was negatively associated with blood control adjusted OR 0.839 (0.742-0.949)	A

Comparison of Quality of Care in VA and Non-VA Settings

Author; Year	Category	VA Sample Data Level	VA Sample Size	VA Years Collected	Non-VA Data Level	Non-VA Sample Size	Non-VA Years Collected	Conditions	Outcomes	Primary Findings	Final Grade
Reiber, G.E., et al.; 2004[39]	Diabetes	Nat'l	535	2000	Nat'l	1848/9055	2000	DM, Preventive care	a1c testings, foot exam, diabetes education, bp measurement, cholesterol measurement, sigmoidoscop, fotb testing among patients with diabetes	Veterans who use VA have higher rates of foot exams, diabetes education, and sigmoidoscopy an da lower rate of a1c testing compared to veterans who did not use the VA. There were non-significatn difference for eye exams, bp measurements, cholestestorol testing and fobt screening.	A
Ritchie, J.L., et al.; 1998[48]	Cardiovascular	One VISN	8326	1993-1994	Lrg geo area	6666	1993-1994	IHD	10 and 30 day mortality, 10 and 30 day use of cardiac bypass surgery	Overall mortality and same-admission bypass surgery rates were similar for patients undergoing PTCA in the VA and Washington State hospitals.	B
Rosenheck, R.A., et al.; 2000[57]	Mental health	Mult ctrs	192/274	1994-1996	Mult ctrs	96/184	1994-1996	Psychosis/schizophrenia	adherence to port recommendations	On 5 of 26 Schizophrenic Patient Outcomes Research Team treatment recommendations, a smaller proportion of VA than non-VA patients adhered to standards. Four of these reflected reduced access among VA patients to psychosocial services such as work therapy, job training, or case management services.	B
Rosenthal, G.E., et al.; 2003[60]	Hospital and nursing home care	Single ctr	1960	1994-1995	Mult ctrs	157147	1994-1995	Other medical/nonsurgical condition	mortality	Risk adjusted inhospital mortality was similar for VA and private sector patients OR 1.07 95%CI 0.74-1.54.	B

Comparison of Quality of Care in VA and Non-VA Settings

Author; Year	Category	VA Sample			Non-VA Sample			Conditions	Outcomes	Primary Findings	Final Grade
		Data Level	Sample Size	Years Collected	Data Level	Sample Size	Years Collected				
Ross, J.S., et al.; 2008[40]	General, mult conditions	Nat'l	10007	2000-2004	Nat'l	393873	2000-2004	DM, IHD, HTN, Preventive Care	self reported use of 17 recommended health care services including cancer prevention, cardiovascular risk reduction, diabetes management and infection prevention.	VAMC care was associated with greater use of recommended services in both years of study (6/17 services more used in 2000, 12/17 more used in 2004)	B
Selim, A.J., et al.; 2006[41]	General, mortality and health status	Nat'l	420514/ 1.5m	1999-2004	Nat'l	584294/ 879202	1998-2004	Other medical/ nonsurgical condition	Risk adjusted mortality	After adjusting for case-mix, the HR for mortality in the MAP was significantly higher than that in the VA (HR, 1.404; 95% CI _ 1.383–1.426).	B
Selim, A.J., et al.; 2007[42]	General, mortality and health status	Nat'l	12177/ 16725	1998-2000	Nat'l	26225/ 62614	1998-2000	None	Risk-adjusted 2 year mortality, change in physical and mental health status	Higher risk-adjusted mortality in the VA compared to Medicare Advantage (2 year mortality 7.6% in VA vs. 9.2% in MA); There were no significant differences in the probability of being alive with the same or better PCS except for the South (VA 65.8% vs. MAP 62.5%, P = .0014).VA patients had a slightly higher probability of being alive with the same or better MCS (71.8% vs. 70.1%, P = .002)	B

Comparison of Quality of Care in VA and Non-VA Settings

Author; Year	Category	VA Sample Data Level	VA Sample Size	VA Years Collected	Non-VA Data Level	Non-VA Sample Size	Non-VA Years Collected	Conditions	Outcomes	Primary Findings	Final Grade
Selim, A.J., et al.; 2009[46]	General, mortality and health status	Nat'l	2361	1999-2000	Nat'l	1912	1999-2000	Other medical/ nonsurgical condition	3 year risk adjusted mortality rate	The adjusted HR of mortality in the MA dual enrollees was significantly higher than in the VHA dual enrollees (HR, 1.260 [95% CI, 1.044–1.520]).	B
Stineman, M.G., et al.; 2001[58]	Other	Nat'l	3056	1994-1995	Nat'l	52382	1995	TIA/Stroke	functional independence	Stroke patients receiving rehabil-itation in the VA setting were discharged with slightly better functional outcomes.	B
Weeks, W.B., et al.; 2008[43]	Hospital and nursing home care	One VISN	105026	1998-2000	Lrg geo	163853	1998-2000	None	length of stay, readmission within 30 days	Across conditions, the length of stay was longer for VA patients compared with non-VA patients. In logistic regression, VA care was not a significant predictor of 30day readmission for veterans <65years old, however for veterans >=65 years of age initial VA admission was associated with a significantly higher odds of readmission within 30 days than non-VA index admission (OR2.79, 95%CI 1.4-5.6)	B
Weeks, W.B., et al.; 2008[44]	Hospital and nursing home care	One VISN	50429	1998-2000	Lrg geo	74017	1998-2000	Patient Safety Indicators	Risk adjusted rates of non-obstetric patient safety indicators	Rates similar for 9 of 15 PSIs, ulcer, sepsis, iatrogenic infection, postop resp failure, post op metabolic derangement lower in VA, mortality higher in VA for low-risk DRGs	B

Comparison of Quality of Care in VA and Non-VA Settings

Author; Year	Category	VA Sample			Non-VA Sample			Conditions	Outcomes	Primary Findings	Final Grade
		Data Level	Sample Size	Years Collected	Data Level	Sample Size	Years Collected				
Wright, S.M., et al.; 1999[49]	Cardio-vascular	Nat'l	14853	1992-1995	Nat'l	32745	1992-1995	IHD	30 day and 1 year adjusted mortality rates	After adjusting for patient characteristics, the odds of 30-day mortality were not significantly different between patients admitted to VA basic service hospitals (reference) and patients admitted to any other type of hospital within either system of care. The odds of 1-year mortality were significantly lower in patients admitted to Medi-care cardiac surgery hospitals (OR 0.88, 95% CI 0.79-0.98) compared to patients admitted to VA basic service hospitals	B

APPENDIX 3. SCREENER FORM

Article ID:_____ Reviewer:_____
First Author:_____
              (Last Name Only)

Study Number: ___of____ Description:_____
         (Enter '1of 1' if only one)   (if more than one study)

1. Does the paper present a comparison of quality of clinical data in VA and US non-VA settings?
Yes..☐
No...☐

If No→ Stop

[NB: exclude the following: pure utilization rates, rates of disease, efficiency, recruitment techniques, and lack of direct comparisons]

2. Are the data for the comparison sufficiently contemporaneous (within 1 to 2 years)?
Yes..☐
No...☐

3. How are the VA data assembled (within sites)?
Random/representative sampling..................☐
Convenience sampling............................☐
Other (specify_____)................☐

4. How are the non-VA data assembled (within sites)?
Random/representative sampling..................☐
Convenience sampling............................☐
Other (specify_____)................☐

5. At what level do the VA data come from?
National or sufficiently multisite
to represent national data......................☐
Multiple VISNs..................................☐
One VISN (or state).............................☐
Multiple medical centers or clinics.............☐
Single medical center or clinic.................☐
Unknown...☐

6. At what level do the non-VA data come from?
National or sufficiently
representative..................................☐
Large geographic area like a state..............☐
Multiple centers or clinics.....................☐
Single medical center or clinic.................☐

7. What conditions are covered by the quality assessment (check all that apply)

Medical and Non-Surgical Quality Areas
CHF..☐
DM...☐
IHD...☐
HTN..☐
Pulmonary Disease......................................☐
Preventive Care..☐
Cancer (list type)...☐
Osteoarthritis..☐
Depression..☐
Psychosis/schizophrenia..............................☐
PTSD..☐
TIA/Stroke..☐
Other (specify_____)......................☐

Surgical Quality Areas
General...☐
Cardiothoracic..☐
Head and Neck...☐
Orthopedic..☐
Surgical Oncology..☐
Urology..☐
Vascular...☐
Other surgical...☐
Other (specify_____)......................☐

Safety Areas
Patient Safety Indicators............................☐
Other (specify_____)......................☐

8. What features of quality are measured?
Structure..☐
Process ....☐
Outcomes ....☐
Structure includes presence/absence of facilities
Process includes overuse, underuse, misuse
Outcomes includes intermediate outcomes

9. How did the specifications for the quality assessments compare in VA and non VA samples?
Identical...☐
Sufficiently similar for valid comparison......☐
Sufficiently dissimilar to present a
threat to valid comparison..........................☐
Unclear...☐

APPENDIX 4. DATA ABSTRACTION FORM

Data Abstraction Form: Round Two

Article ID: <<Pre-filled from database>>
Reviewer: <<Pre-filled from database>>
Author/ Year: <<Pre-filled from database>>
VA sample: <<Pre-filled from database>> (random/rep, convenience AND national, multisite, etc.)
Non-VA sample: <<Pre-filled from database>> (same two sets of information)
Conditions: <<Pre-filled from database>>

Sample size used
    VA:
    Non-VA:
Years of data collection covered
    VA:
    Non-VA:
Control variables:
Primary outcomes:
Findings (adjusted if possible):
Secondary/associated findings (optional):
Assessment (grade each of the following with A/B/C scale):
    ___1. Time frames
    ___2. Samples (both VA and non-VA)
    ___3. Quality measurements
    ___4. Outcomes
    ___5. Importance of measures
    ___6. Statistical methods
Other/notes:
Overall assessment/assignment of level:
Rejected (Graded C or lower, or failed to meet prior criteria):

APPENDIX 5. DATA ABSTRACTION GRADING GUIDELINES

Assessment (grade levels detailed below):
1. Time frames
    A. Contemporaneous time frames
    B. All between A and C
    C. non-contemporaneous
2. Samples (both VA and non-VA)
    A. representative or national samples (both VA and non-VA)
    B. All between A and C
    C. small, limited, unequal or non-representative samples
3. Quality measurements
    A. specified and identical measures with a similar assessment format for those measures
    B. All between A and C
    C. dissimilar measures and/or dissimilar assessment methods
4. Outcomes
    A. outcomes are either well established clinical endpoints or processes strongly associated with well-established clinical endpoints
    B. All between A and C
    C. outcomes are structures, processes or clinical endpoints that are not well-established or are indirect measures of quality
5. Importance of measures (e.g. number of clinically relevant indicators, potential impact of indicators)
    A. High
    B. Medium
    C. Low
6. Statistical methods
    A. Sufficient sample size and/or methods appropriate to address hypothesis(ses)
    B. All between A and C
    C. Insufficient sample size and/or methods questionable to address hypothesis(ses)

Overall assessment/assignment of level: Measured as an average of grades assigned above

APPENDIX 6. SEARCH STRATEGY

TOPIC: Veterans Hospitals and Non-Veterans Hospitals Quality of Care – Search Methodology

NOTE: Search strategy was derived from subject terms used in 34 articles provided by the project

Database: PubMed
Years Covered: 1996- 2009 (August)
Number of results: 432

Search Strategy:
hospitals, veterans[MeSH Terms] OR hospitals, veterans[majr] OR hospitals, veterans/standards OR hospitals, veterans/statistics and numerical data OR united states department of veterans affairs OR united states department of veterans affairs/standards OR united states department of veterans affairs/statistics and numerical data OR united states department of veterans affairs/utilization

APPENDIX 7. PEER REVIEW COMMENTS TABLE

Location	Comment	Change
Executive Summary, Background	I am curious about why you do not mention the "Best Care Anywhere" book and others, and only focus upon negative?	Background updated to incorporate suggested citation.
Executive Summary, Conclusion	Might clarify that medication process of care showed VA was better, but procedural process of care not uniformly better (ie angiography).	"…and interventional procedures" added for clarification.
Hospital and Nursing Home Care, Summary	"Racial mortality differences" to "mortality rates for racial minorities"	Change incorporated
Mental Health, Summary	It wasn't clear in the summary how outpatient follow-up rates could be worse when outpatient continuity was better, so I tried to clarify: "…and [timely] outpatient visit follow-up rates [after discharge] were worse in the VA, but continuity of care [in the outpatient setting]…"	Change incorporated
Conclusions, paragraph 9	Same comments as in the mental health section above: "…equivalent racial mortality differences…" to "equivalent mortality rates across racial groups"	Change incorporated

www.ingramcontent.com/pod-product-compliance
Lightning Source LLC
Chambersburg PA
CBHW081614170526
45166CB00009B/2959